J. B. Fiebach P. D. Schellinger Stroke MRI

with K. Sartor S. Heiland S. Warach W. Hacke

JOCHEN B. FIEBACH
PETER D. SCHELLINGER
with
KLAUS SARTOR
SABINE HEILAND
STEVEN WARACH
WERNER HACKE

Stroke MRI

With 47 Figures in 117 Separate Illustrations
and 13 Tables

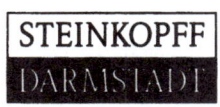

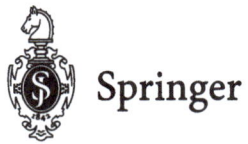

Dr. med. Jochen B. Fiebach
Abteilung Neuroradiologie
Neurologische Klinik
des Universitätsklinikums
Ruprecht-Karls-Universität Heidelberg
Im Neuenheimer Feld 400
69120 Heidelberg

Priv.-Doz. Dr. med. Peter D. Schellinger
Abt. Neurologie und Poliklinik
Neurologische Klinik
der Universität Heidelberg
Ruprecht-Karls-Universität Heidelberg
Im Neuenheimer Feld 400
69120 Heidelberg

Prof. Dr. med. Klaus Sartor
Direktor Abteilung Neuroradiologie
Neurologische Klinik
des Universitätsklinikums
Ruprecht-Karls-Universität Heidelberg
Im Neuenheimer Feld 400
69120 Heidelberg

Priv.-Doz Dr. rer. nat. Sabine Heiland
Abteilung Neuroradiologie
Neurologische Klinik
des Universitätsklinikums
Ruprecht-Karls-Universität Heidelberg
Im Neuenheimer Feld 400
69120 Heidelberg

Steven Warach, MD, PhD
Stroke Diagnostic
and Therapeutic Section
Stroke Branch, NINDS
Building 10, Room B1D733
10 Center Drive, MSC 1063
Bethesda, MD 20892-1063
USA

Prof. Dr. med. Dipl.-Psych. Werner Hacke
Direktor Abt. Neurologie
und Poliklinik
Neurologische Klinik
der Universität Heidelberg
Ruprecht-Karls-Universität Heidelberg
Im Neuenheimer Feld 400
69120 Heidelberg

Additional material to this book can be downloaded from http://extras.springer.com

ISBN 978-3-642-63253-2   ISBN 978-3-642-57387-3 (eBook)
DOI 10.1007/978-3-642-57387-3

Cataloging-in-Publication Data applied for
A catalog record for this book is available from the Library of Congress.
Bibliographic information published by Die Deutsche Bibliothek
Die Deutsche Bibliothek lists this publication in the Deutsche Nationalbibliografie;
detailed bibliographic data is available in the Internet at <http://dnb.ddb.de>.

www.steinkopff.springer.de

© Springer-Verlag Berlin Heidelberg 2003
Originally published by Steinkopff-Verlag Darmstadt in 2003
Softcover reprint of the hardcover 1st edition 2003

The use of general descriptive names, registered names, trademarks, etc. in this publication does not imply, even in the absence of a specific statement, that such names are exempt from the relevant protective laws and regulations and therefore free for general use.

Product liability: The publishers cannot guarantee the accuracy of any information about the application of operative techniques and medications contained in this book. In every individual case the user must check such information by consulting the relevant literature.

Production: Klemens Schwind
Cover Design: Erich Kirchner, Heidelberg
Typesetting: K+V Fotosatz GmbH, Beerfelden

SPIN 10980620   85/7231-5 4 3 2 1 – Printed on acid-free paper

Preface

During the last decade – the decade of the brain – the therapeutic attitude towards stroke therapy and prophylaxis has changed. It has become clear that adequate imaging of stroke is a necessity in order to optimize selection of stroke patients for specific therapies and, thus, improve stroke outcome. While being the standard of care, CT is less sensitive to the different pathophysiological facets we are facing in acute stroke patients where distinct stroke dynamics characterize the individual patient at an individual point in time. The authors present an overview of stroke MR imaging beginning with a review of the technical aspects and current standards of imaging. In the main text, the role of stroke MRI in ischemic stroke and intracranial hemorrhage including subarachnoid hemorrhage as well as trial design are considered. The recommendations for guiding thrombolytic therapy based on stroke MRI findings are our expressed expert opinion but are not necessarily consistent with the regulations imposed by the respective drug administrations or international guidelines. Therefore, we ask the reader of this book to mind the local regulations. Before applying thrombolytic therapy outside an officially accepted protocol or approved indication, local institutional review board approval must be obtained as well as informed consent from the patient or his/her relatives. The book is complemented by a CD-ROM, which in addition to an extensive compilation of imaging data, is a self-assessment and teaching tool that will enable the user to read stroke MRI scans.

Heidelberg, December 2002

JOCHEN B. FIEBACH
PETER D. SCHELLINGER

Contents

Abbreviations

ACA	Anterior Cerebral Artery	MCA	Middle Cerebral Artery
ADC	Apparent Diffusion Coefficient	MRA	Magnetic Resonance Angiography
BBB	Blood Brain Barrier	mRS	modified Rankin Scale
BI	Barthel Index	MRI	Magnetic Resonance Imaging
CBF	Cerebral Blood Flow	MTT	Mean Transit Time $\cong$ Time to passage of 50% of the contrast agent bolus
CBV	Cerebral Blood Volume $\cong$ Area under the Concentration Time Curve		
CSF	Cerebrospinal Fluid	NIHSS	National Institutes of Health Stroke Scale
CT	Computed Tomography	PCA	Posterior Cerebral Artery
CTA	CT Angiography	PCT	Perfusion CT
CTA-SI	CTA Source Images	PD-WI	Proton Density-weighted Imaging
DSA	Digital Subtraction Angiography		
DSC	Dynamic Susceptibility Contrast-enhanced Imaging	PWI	Perfusion-weighted Imaging
		RCT	Randomized Controlled Trial
DWI	Diffusion-weighted Imaging	ROI	Region of Interest
DU	Doppler/Duplex Ultrasound	SAH	Subarachnoid Hemorrhage
EIS	Early Infarct Signs	SE	Spin Echo
EPI	Echo Planar Imaging	S-MRI	Stroke MRI
FLAIR	Fluid Attenuated Inversion Recovery	SWI	Susceptibility-weighted Imaging
FLASH	Fast Low Angle Shot	SSS	Scandinavian Stroke Scale
GE	Gradient Echo	TAR	Tissue at Risk
GOS	Glasgow Outcome Score	T1-WI	T1-weighted Imaging
HMCAS	Hyperdense Middle Cerebral Artery Sign	T2-WI	T2-weighted Imaging
		T2*-WI	T2-"Star"-weighted Imaging $\cong$ SWI
ICA	Internal Carotid Artery		
ICH	Intracerebral Hemorrhage	TTP	Time to Peak = Time to maximum arrival of the contrast agent bolus
IS	Ischemic Stroke		

1 Introduction

J. B. Fiebach, P. D. Schellinger

Stroke is the third leading cause of death after myocardial infarction and cancer and the leading cause of permanent disability in western countries [386, 387]. Furthermore, it is the leading cause of disability adjusted loss of independent life years. Aside from the tragic consequences for the patients and their families, the socio-economic impact of more or less disabled stroke survivors is evident as stroke patients with permanent deficits such as hemiparesis and aphasia will frequently not be able to live independently or pursue an occupation. The added indirect and direct cost estimates for a survived stroke vary between 35000 and 50000 US$ per year. In the face of our aging population and the skewed population pyramid, the incidence and prevalence of stroke is expected to rise. Therefore, an effective treatment for this devastating disease is desperately needed. However, for a long time acute stroke has been a disease without specific therapeutic options. In general, therapy consisted of medical stabilization in the acute setting and, eventually, adjustment of risk factors. Formerly, but in many countries even today, stroke patients are treated in general internal medicine wards and not by specialists or stroke neurologists. In many countries CT imaging is not routinely performed. Most therapies for acute stroke that have been formally tested in double blinded randomized controlled trials yielded negative results. This includes plasma expanders, anticoagulation, neuroprotectants, and free radical scavengers. The rather nihilistic approach to treating stroke has changed during the last decade as several studies have shown the efficacy of recanalizing drugs and promising results for single neuroprotectants in acute ischemic stroke patients. Under these circumstances, neuroradiology with its new imaging modalities has become a major player in the diagnostic workup of, but also in the therapeutic approach to acute stroke patients. However, not only for stroke specialists but also for the neuroradiologist, it has become essential to understand the pathophysiology of stroke beyond the technology of their diagnostic tools. With a growing knowledge on the neuroradiologist's part and new techniques available, the neuroradiologist becomes an equal partner in the diagnostic and therapeutic discussion.

The target for most therapeutic interventions for focal ischemia should be ischemic tissue that can respond to treatment and is not irreversibly injured. Such tissue will be defined as potentially salvageable ischemic tissue and must be distinguished from nonsalvageable ischemic tissue, that has evolved to a status, in which recovery is no longer possible. The characterization of potentially reversible versus irreversible loss of function is based on the concept of the ischemic penumbra. Until recently only PET and SPECT imaging could approximately define ischemia and penumbra thresholds. This is however not feasible for caregivers in a broad population, where imaging in an acute setting is confined to CT and also increasingly MR imaging. Only the advent of new imaging techniques such as novel sequences and continuing improvement of imaging hardware allows an improvement in the diagnostic yield. An adequate therapy demands an adequate diagnostic workup first. In the following chapters we will introduce the reader to the current state of stroke imaging with a focus on new MR imaging techniques, but we will also cover current imaging standards such as CT and evolving alternative CT techniques. In the face of recanalization therapies, the only therapy so far proven to be effective, a special emphasis is laid on MRI features in these patients including the theoretic background, practical issues such as procedural algorithms, differential diagnosis of ischemic and hemorrhagic stroke as well as an overview of thrombolysis. The final chapters deal with future perspectives with regard to imaging but also trial design as stroke MRI may be used to guide inclusion or exclusion of patients into randomized controlled trials based on imaging findings. Together with the case collection and self-assessment feature on the accompanying CD-ROM, the reader will be able to interpret stroke MRI findings and guide therapeutic management based on understanding of advantages and limitations of the diagnostic tool.

2 CT as the Current Standard in Stroke Imaging

P.D. Schellinger, J.B. Fiebach, W. Hacke

Non-contrast CT imaging is the current diagnostic standard for stroke imaging [159] mainly due to its close to 100% high sensitivity for intracerebral hemorrhage (ICH), which is the most important differential diagnosis for ischemic stroke [364]. A standard CT protocol includes axial CT scanning with a slice thickness of 3–5 mm for the posterior fossa and 8–10 mm for suprasellar structures. Indeed the differentiation of ischemic stroke and ICH by clinical means alone is impossible. Although early deterioration of vigilance, vomiting in anterior circulation as opposed to posterior circulation syndrome, coumadine therapy, or a hypertensive crisis may hint towards ICH, these symptoms can also be seen in ischemic stroke. Mainly in the early 1990s and based on the CT images collected in thrombolysis trials, an effort was made to also define early signs of ischemic infarction on CT scans. However, there is the still widely held false belief that early CT (within the first hours) is insensitive to changes after ischemic stroke. Even in newer textbooks or in recent papers in high-rated non-neuroradiological journals, it is considered that CT is negative with regard to ischemic tissue changes during the first 12 hours after symptom onset [106, 107]. However, during the last few years it has been generally accepted in the neuroradiological community that CT can demonstrate early infarct signs within the first 6 hours after stroke. With the availability of high-quality CT scanners more and more investigators reported their positive CT-findings in early ischemic stroke. The sensitivity of these findings varies widely ranging from 12% to 92%, depending on the infarct signs, the exact time window of the investigated population, and on the authors.

The most common sign of an early infarct is a gray matter hypodensity, which develops in the early stages of an infarction and can be subtle, and thus difficult to detect. The development of an extracellular edema can be recognized even during the first few hours after stroke onset and is due to a masking of cortical or deep nuclear structures. This phenomenon can be demonstrated best in cases of an acute occlusion of the main stem of the middle cerebral artery (M1 occlusion), where the parenchymal hypodensity can be identified first in terminal artery supply areas, like the basal ganglia [36, 364, 369]. Depending on the origin of the recurrent artery of Heubner this hypodensity also involves the head of the caudate nucleus. In cases with insufficient leptomeningeal collaterals the primary hypodensity involves cortical structures, i.e., the insula, known as the „loss of the insular ribbon sign" [345], or other territories of the middle cerebral artery.

The incidence of hypodensities in patients with acute stroke is reported over a wide range and certainly depends on the percent of patients with a major vessel occlusion (i.e., M1-segment). More recent studies have reported incidences of early CT signs of infarction between 53% and 92% within the first 6 hours for all acute stroke patients [154, 343, 364, 368]. In patients with a M1-segment occlusion, the incidence of a parenchymal hypodensity is reported with 68% within the first two hours but increases to 89% in the third hour after symptom onset and up to 100% thereafter [368]. A reversibility of this early hypodensity has not been reported, though there is a correlation between the size of early hypodensities and the risk of a secondary hemorrhage [35] and clinical outcome. Von Kummer showed that early parenchymal hypodensity covering more than an estimated 50% of the MCA territory is a specific finding associated with a mortality of 85% [368]. The same findings could be confirmed by the ECASS trial: mortality was 13% in patients without hypodensity, 23% in patients with parenchymal hypodensity less than 33% of the MCA territory, and 49% in patients with an early hypodensity exceeding 33% of the MCA territory [125]. Confirmed by both, ECASS trials I and II, it has been clearly shown that the clinical response to intravenous rt-PA in patients with ischemic stroke can be predicted on the basis of initial CT findings. These studies showed that in patients with a small area of hypoattenuation (<33% of the MCA territory), treatment increased the chance of a good clinical outcome. In patients with a normal baseline CT scan or in patients with a large area of hypoattenuation (>33% of the MCA territory), rt-PA had no benefit but increased the risk for a fatal brain hemorrhage [361]. Focal brain swelling of the ischemic territory leads to a sulcal effacement, which can be recognized best by direct comparison of the two hemispheres (Fig. 2.1). Although severe brain swelling occurs more in the acute (12 to 24 hours) or subacute (>24 hours) stage of an ischemia, it can also be demonstrated within the first 6 hours after stroke in 12% to 41% of stroke patients [154, 364]. The hyperdense middle cerebral artery sign (HMCAS) as seen on unenhanced CT is defined as a part of the MCA being denser than other parts of the vessel or its counterpart not attributable to calcification [341, 342]. This sign describes the visualization of the thrombus itself within the vessel and can also be noted in other vessels of the circle of Willis. The HMCAS is present in 40–60% of patients with angiographically proven MCA occlusion of any type [202, 342, 368]. In a primarily unselected population of stroke patients, the HMCAS was found in about 17%, but was associated with severe brain ischemia and poor clinical outcome [212]. Nevertheless, the same study showed that patients with an HMCAS may benefit from thrombolysis when they do not show a large hypodensity in the initial CT scan (Fig. 2.2).

Intravenous thrombolytic therapy with rt-PA presently requires documentation of an acute onset focal neurological deficit with a baseline NIHSS score [208], adhering to general blood pressure guidelines, accounting

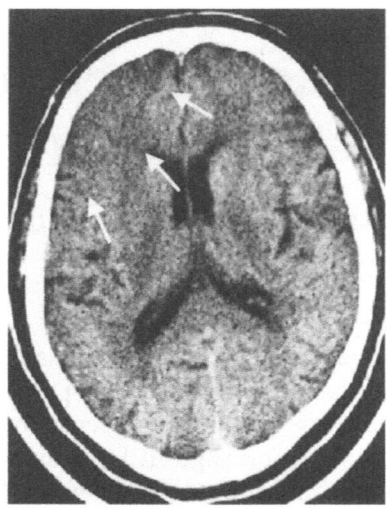

Fig. 2.1. Non-contrast CT scan with a right frontal hypodensity of less than one-third of the MCA territory, sulcal effacement on loss of differentiation of cortical gray and white matter (*see arrows*)

for general rt-PA-contraindications, and exclusion of ICH by CT. These are the criteria by which rt-PA was proven effective within 3 h in the NINDS trial in 1995 and FDA approved in 1996 [338]. We believe, however, that these are the absolute minimum requirements which are not in keeping with times and therefore should be extended by one or several of the following: the ECASS CT criteria define early signs of ischemic infarction (EIS) that improve infarct detection and estimation of actual infarct size [364, 369]. The most common EIS are a subtle deep gray matter and/or cortical hypodensity, loss of the insular ribbon, sulcal effacement due to early edema and the hyperdense middle cerebral artery sign [364] (Fig. 2.3, Fig. 2.4). While several studies have shown the usefulness of early CT findings to select patients before intravenous thrombolytic therapy, other studies demonstrated that physicians including general radiologists and neurologists do not uniformly achieve a sufficient level of sensitivity for identification of CT contraindications for thrombolytic therapy (i.e., intracerebral hemorrhage or early signs of ischemia) [312]. However, the recognition of early infarct signs by CT can be trained and the positive effect of training in reading CT scans of hyperacute stroke patients has been shown in a large trial [360]. A post hoc

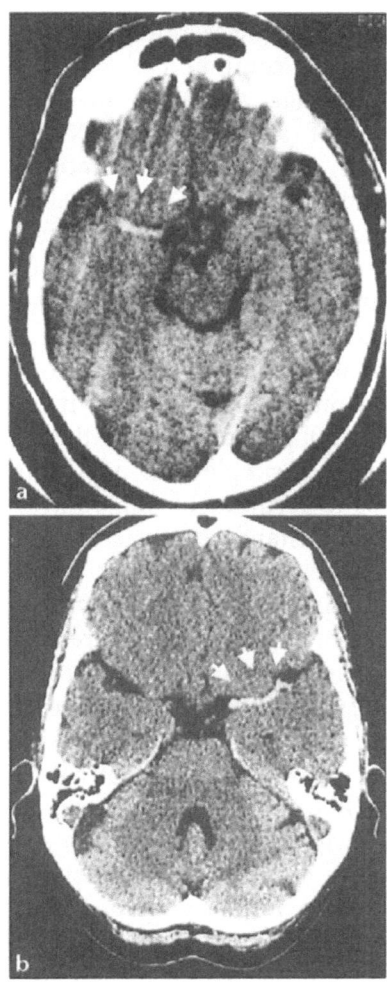

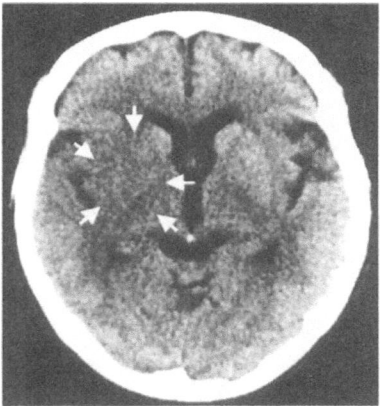

Fig. 2.3. Non-contrast CT scan with loss of basal ganglia differentiation on the right side. Compared to the normal left side thalamus and putamen are hypodense (*arrows*)

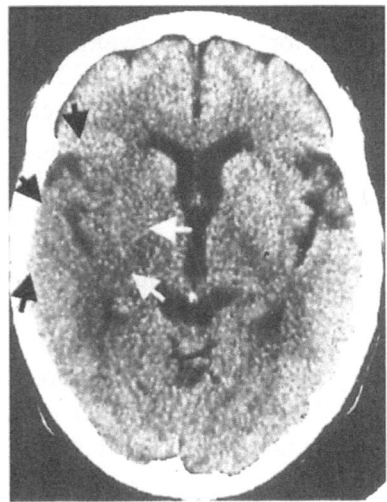

Fig. 2.2. Non-contrast CT scan with a hyperdense MCA sign on the right (**a**) and on the left (**b**). Arrowheads depict the intravascular thrombus as a high signal

Fig. 2.4. Non-contrast CT scan. Loss of the insular ribbon (*arrows*)

analysis of the NINDS CT data (N=616) yielded a 31% sensitivity for EIS, a mild correlation with the acute NIHSS score but neither an effect on clinical outcome nor on secondary ICH rate [262]. However, it was not assessed whether outcome would have been better if rt-PA had not been given to patients with EIS >33% of the MCA territory. Furthermore, these criteria apply more to patients in the 3–6 h time window (ECASS I and II) as many CT scans are negative within the first 2 h. Therefore, patients with early signs of infarction/demarcation exceeding one third of the MCA territory should not be treated if no other information is at hand. Among stroke experts, there is consensus that signs

of profound ischemia with a strong hypodensity should not be given rt-PA even within the 3 h time window because of an excessive risk of ICH (Fig. 2.5). Subtle EIS might not definitely develop into infarction; therefore they may be partially reversible and, at least in the 3 h time window, may not be correlated with efficacy of thrombolytic therapy or outcome. In conclusion the established role of non-contrast CT with regard to therapeutic decision making, as agreed upon by the NINDS and ECASS groups, is the exclusion of ICH and the exclusion of patients with extensive demarcation of ischemic infarctions.

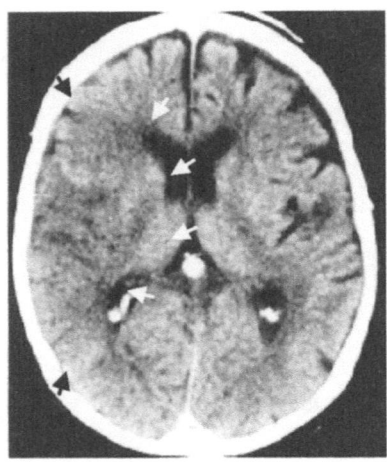

Fig. 2.5. Non-contrast CT scan with an early hypodensity of approximately two-thirds of the right MCA territory including the putamen and sparing the thalamus (*arrows*)

A new instrument for the improvement of the CT rating is the ASPECTS score [20, 264]. The ASPECTS score divides the middle-cerebral-artery territory into ten regions of interest as seen on two standardized axial CT slices (basal ganglia and lateral ventricles). The whole MCA territory is allotted 10 points (one for each area) and a single point is subtracted for each of the defined regions if ischemic lesions are seen. Interrater variability (Kappa) statistics showed that the interobserver reliability of ASPECTS was higher than that of the 1/3 MCA rule although other pre-liminary data contradict these findings (Werner Hacke, personal communication). The baseline ASPECTS value correlated inversely with the severity of stroke on the NIHSS ($r = -0.56$, $p < 0.001$) and predicted functional outcome and symptomatic ICH ($p < 0.001$; $p = 0.012$). A sharp increase in dependence and death occurs with an ASPECTS score of 7 or less. While the ASPECTS score may be superior to the ECASS 1/3 MCA rule, it is rather a refinement of that rule than a completely new development. Furthermore, it has not been validated for patients outside the 3 h time window. Another simple method to improve the diagnostic accuracy of non-contrast CT is the use of nonstandard, variable window width and level review settings [198]. With standard viewing parameters, sensitivity and specificity for stroke detection were 57% and 100%, with narrow window and variable settings sensitivity significantly increased to 71% without loss of specificity ($p = 0.03$). In conclusion, the sensitivity of non-contrast CT for ICH is high. While clearly defined, the diagnostic impact of early infarct signs is debatable as these signs may often be subtle and require a high level of experience for detection and interpretation. A large area of manifest hypodensity exceeding one-third of the MCA territory, however, should be regarded as a contraindication for thrombolytic therapy.

3 Stroke Scales

P. D. Schellinger

While the assessment of stroke patients and severity grading as well as grading of clinical outcome is not a primary topic of this book, we use the following scales quite frequently and therefore want to supply the reader not familiar with these tools an overview of stroke and outcome scales; for the single scales we refer to Tables 3.1–3.6. The assessment and interpretation of clinical signs with scales and scores is an important part of the diagnostic workup of patients. Scales in general aim to attribute a number (score) to grade or describe a specific clinical syndrome. In most instances, this is an ordinal scale with a rank system. The intervals between different scores are not identical, which implies that non-parametric statistical tests have to be used, which is frequently disregarded in publications, even in highly ranked journals. Also for these scales, median instead of mean values must be used; for instance, a stroke patient with a NIHSS score of 4 is not twice as sick as a patient with a NIHSS score of 2 [73, 354]. Assessment or quantification of biological parameters takes place on four different levels: biological activity (laboratory data, physiological tests, radiological tests), clinical manifestation (degree of severity), function (extent of disability), and quality of life (handicap scales, questionnaires). Most complex scales and scores follow an additive principle, i.e., they consist of subscores that categorize a specific symptom (e.g., different grades of hemiparesis). Each category has a numerical value, and the subscores are added to obtain the final score. These clinical scores to assess disease (e.g., stroke) severity do not necessarily reflect function [115]. A stroke patient with a dense hemisensory deficit and a facial nerve palsy may have the same score as a patient with hemiparesis or aphasia. Stroke scales may be suitable to describe initial or acute stroke severity but are not the ideal tool to assess functional outcome or level of independence. Furthermore, scores and scales do not differentiate on the individual level, e.g., a low grade left-sided arm paresis has other implications for a pianist than possibly for another profession. Disease severity from the patient's view is another important dimension [320].

The stroke scale most widely used today is the National Institutes of Health Stroke Scale (NIHSS) [44]. The NIHSS (Table 3.1) tests several items such as paresis, aphasia, level of consciousness, sensory symptoms, facial and gaze palsy, dysarthria and hemineglect. It has good interrater reliability and excellent validity, which can be further increased by video-assisted training and self-assessment [208]. Two potential disadvantages are a ceiling effect and a bias towards higher scores in left hemispheric infarctions. The score ranges from 0 (no symptoms) to 42 (maximum points in all categories); death is not coded. The Scandinavian Stroke Scale (SSS; Table 3.2) contains 9 items (consciousness, eye movements, strength of arm, hand and leg, orientation, speech, facial palsy and gait) [277, 299]. The score ranges from 0 (maximum deficit) to 56 (no deficits). Patients with a consciousness level below somnolence are not well described with the SSS. The SSS has good interrater reliability and moderate sensitivity. Crossed comparison with other scales showed a good validity. The Glasgow coma scale (GCS; Table 3.3) is the most common tool used for the assessment of reduced consciousness [331]. It is widely distributed, has high validity and reliability, is easy to apply and its use does not imply special medical knowledge. The GCS was originally designed for patients with traumatic brain injury but can be used in coma patients with any other etiology as well.

Table 3.1. National Institutes of Health Stroke Scale (NIHSS)

Item	Factor	Score
Level of consciousness (LOC)	Alert, keenly responsive	0
	Drowsy, but arousable	1
	Requires repeated and strong stimulation to attend or make movements (not stereotyped), lethargic or obtundent	2
	Reflex motor or autonomic effects only, flaccid, reflexless	3
Level of consciousness questions (patient age and actual month)	Answers both correctly	0
	Answers one correctly	1
	Answers both incorrectly or is not able to speak	2
Level of consciousness commands (open and/or close eyes, press hands)	Obeys both correctly	0
	Obeys one correctly	1
	Incorrect	2
Extraocular movements	Normal	0
	Partial gaze palsy	1
	Forced eye deviation, total gaze paresis not overcome by OCR	2
Visual fields	No visual loss	0
	Partial hemianopia	1
	Complete hemianopia 1 side	2
	Complete hemianopia bilateral	3
Facial palsy	Normal	0
	Minor	1
	Partial	2
	Complete	3
Motor arm	Limb holds 90° for 10 s	0
	Limb holds 90° for less than 10 s	1
	Limb cannot hold 90°, some effort against gravity	2
	Limb falls, no effort against gravity but innervation	3
	Plegia	4
Motor leg	Limb holds 30° for 5 s	0
	Limb holds 30° for less than 5 s	1
	Limb cannot hold 30°, some effort against gravity	2
	Limb falls, no effort against gravity	3
	Plegia	4
Limb ataxia	Absent	0
	Present in one limb	1
	Present in two limbs	2
Sensory	Normal, no sensory loss	0
	Mild to moderate sensory loss	1
	Severe to total sensory loss	2
Neglect	No neglect	0
	Visual, auditory or tactile hemi-inattention	1
	Profound inattention to more than one modality	2
Dysarthria	Normal	0
	Mild to moderate, can be understood with difficulty	1
	Severe, unintelligible	2
Language	Normal	0
	Mild to moderate with paraphasias, naming errors, word finding errors	1
	Severe, fully developed Broca's- or Wernicke's-aphasia	2
	Mute or global aphasia	3

Table 3.2. Scandinavian Stroke Scale (SSS)

1. **Level of consciousness (LOC)**	Awake/oriented	6
	Somnolent but oriented	4
	Soporous/not oriented	2
2. **Gaze palsy**	None	4
	Partial	2
	Fixed/complete	0
3. **Paresis upper limb**	MRC 5/5	6
	MRC 4/5	5
	MRC 3/5	4
	MRC 2/5	2
	MRC 0-1/5	0
4. **Paresis hand**	MRC 5/5	6
	MRC 4/5, full range	4
	MRC 2-3/5, finger does not reach hand	2
	MRC 0-1/5	0
5. **Paresis lower limb**	MRC 5/5	6
	MRC 4/5	5
	MRC 3/5	4
	MRC 2/5	2
	MRC 0-1/5	0
6. **LOC questions**	Person, time and location	6
	Two of three	4
	One of three	2
	Completely desoriented	0
7. **Speech**	None	10
	Mild aphasia	6
	No sentences, more than Yes/no	3
	Yes/no or less	0
8. **Facial palsy**	None	2
	Present	0
9. **Walk**	Walk 5 m without assistance	12
	Walk with aid (stick, crutch)	9
	Walk with aid of another person	6
	Sit without help	3
	Bedridden	0

Table 3.3. Glasgow Coma Scale (GCS)

Item	Factor	Score
Best motor response	Obeys	6
	Localizes	5
	Withdraws (flexion)	4
	Abnormal flexion	3
	Extensor response	2
	Nil	1
Verbal response	Oriented	5
	Confused conversation	4
	Inappropriate words	3
	Incomprehensible sounds	2
	Nil	1
Eye opening	Spontaneous	4
	To speech	3
	To pain	2
	Nil	1

The three most common outcome scores for stroke patients are the Barthel index (BI, Table 3.4), the modified Rankin Scale (mRS; Table 3.5) and the Glasgow outcome scale (GOS; Table 3.6) [163, 211, 272, 330]. The GOS scale is predominantly a scale for outcome assessment after traumatic brain injury with low sensitivity. Furthermore, it has only one category that describes a functional pa-

tient (GOS 5), whereas scores 2–4 describe various degrees of incapacitation. The BI assesses ten functions of daily life such as dressing, bladder and bowel function, personal toilet, ascend and descend stairs, bathing, etc. It is an easy to handle instrument and does not need any special training. It has good reliability and validity with a moderate sensitivity. One further advantage is that the BI score can be assessed via a telephone interview (as opposed to the NIHSS or SSS). The mRS is a very simple scale to assess outcome after ischemic stroke. The score ranges from 0 (no symptoms at all) to 6 (death), can also be assessed via telephone interviews and allows a good dichotomization into favorable (scores 0–1) versus unfavorable (scores 2–6) or independent (scores 0–2) versus dependent or dead (scores 3–6) outcome. A BI of 95 or 100 points is usually considered to be a good outcome; some trials assess a combined endpoint such as BI≥95 and mRS 0 or 1. Stroke scales are frequently used to determine early improvement such as NIHSS score reduction of 7 or more points within 24 hours. More recently, a graded response system has been proposed and validated in a large Phase IIb study (AbBEST) (unpublished data). In this system, successful therapy was defined depending on initial stroke severity. For example, a patient with a NIHSS score of 3 will most likely have a mRS score of 0 after three

Table 3.4. Barthel Index (BI)

1. Eat	Without help	10
	With little help (e.g. cutting)	5
	Fully dependent	0
2. Transfer from bed to wheelchair	Independent	15
	Needs minimal help	10
	Cannot sit up in bed, has to be lifted from the bed but can help	5
	Fully dependent	0
3. Grooming	Independent	5
	Fully dependent	0
4. Toilet use	Fully independent	10
	Needs some help (e.g. toilet paper, balance)	5
	Fully dependent	0
5. Use of shower and bath	Independent	5
	Fully dependent	0
6. Walk 50 m on a horizontal path, may use stick but not a walker	Independent with aids (e.g. stick, crutches)	15
	with aid of a person	10
	Independent with wheelchair	5
	Fully dependent	0
7. Walk stairs, may use stick or crutches	Independent	10
	Needs help	5
	Fully dependent	0
8. Dressing	Independent	10
	Needs help (can do >50% alone)	5
	Fully dependent	0
9. Bowel continence (includes self-management of stoma)	Independent, no accidents	10
	Partially incontinent	5
	Completely incontinent	0
10. Urinary continence (includes self-management of catheter)	Independent, no accidents	10
	Partially incontinent	5
	Completely incontinent	0

Table 3.5. The modified Rankin Scale (mRS)

Grade 0	No symptoms
Grade 1	Residual symptoms but full function, can perform all duties and tasks of daily life
Grade 2	Mild impairment, cannot perform all tasks as before but fully independent
Grade 3	Moderate impairment, needs some help but can walk
Grade 4	Moderate to severe impairment, cannot walk without help, needs help on a regular base
Grade 5	Severely disabled, bedridden, continuous help and nursing required.
Grade 6	Death

0–1 Good outcome
0–2 Independent outcome

Table 3.6. Glasgow Outcome Scale (GOS)

Grade 1	Death
Grade 2	Persistent vegetative state
Grade 3	Severely disabled, continuous help and nursing required
Grade 4	Moderate impairment
Grade 5	No or minimal impairment only

months, meaning that a mRS score of 0 or 1 is not necessarily proof of successful treatment. On the other hand, a patient with a baseline NIHSS score of 15 points or more is very successfully treated, if the 3 month mRS score is 2.

In conclusion, stroke and outcome scales are a useful tool to assess stroke severity and functional outcome with a numerical score that to a certain extent allows categorization of patients and, with regard to stroke imaging, allows the correlation of clinical findings with imaging results.

4 Conventional MRI, Diffusion-weighted MRI (DWI) and Apparent Diffusion Coefficient (ADC)

J. B. FIEBACH, P. D. SCHELLINGER, S. HEILAND, K. SARTOR

Aside from the new MR imaging techniques, a stroke MRI protocol consists at least in part of conventional or standard MR sequences such as T1-WI, T2-WI, FLAIR and MRA. On T2-WI ischemic infarction appears as a hyperintense lesion (Fig. 4.1).

Definite signal changes, however, are at the earliest seen 2 hours after stroke onset in animal experiments and 6–8 hours after stroke onset in human stroke [74, 226, 381, 392]. Neither a diagnosis of parenchymal ischemia nor the differentiation of ischemic core from penumbral tissue is possible with T2-WI [317]. Only when water diffuses into the extracellular space as a consequence of blood brain barrier (BBB) breakdown, i. e., vasogenic edema, will a significant increase of the T2-relaxation time lead to a signal increase on T2-WI which persists throughout the process of tissue necrotization and resorption into the chronic stage of infarction. However, it has been shown by correlation with definitive hypodensities on CT that T2-WI lesions in ischemic stroke patients correlate well with tissue prognosis [384].

On T1-WI an early infarction is characterized by focal swelling and parenchymal hypointensity (Fig. 4.2) due to cytotoxic edema with a T1-time increase and vascular enhancement after administration of gadolinium contrast agent due to hypoperfusion and residual intravascular contrast agent [48, 153, 392]. These signs, however, are not reliable or sensitive during the first hours after stroke onset and can also be a sign in higher grade vessel stenosis [74, 239]. In the subacute stage there may be parenchymal enhancement in postcontrast images after BBB breakdown, which is associated with outcome, where early and more intense enhancement is correlated with a better clinical outcome as opposed to late and progressive enhancement [74].

The Fluid Attenuated Inversion-Recovery (FLAIR) technique results in strongly T2-WI with selective suppression of the CSF signal al-

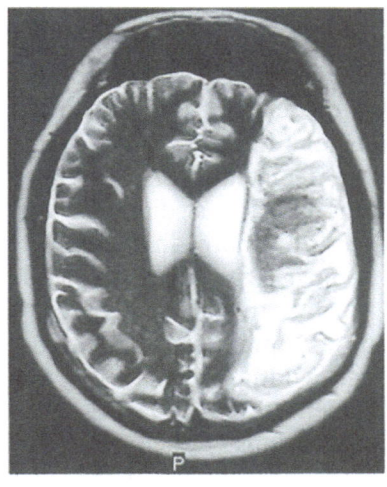

Fig. 4.1. T2-WI shows a subacute ischemic infarction of the entire MCA territory on the left side. There is an area of hypointensity due to hemorrhagic transformation within the infarct. This signal loss is caused by susceptibility artifacts due to blood degradation products

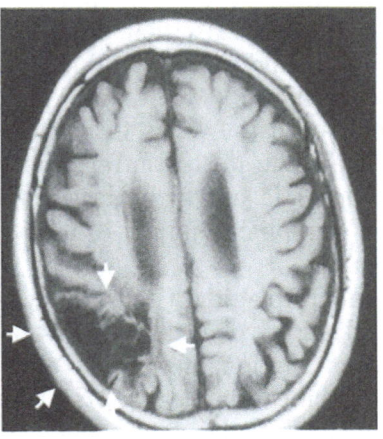

Fig. 4.2. T1-WI shows an old embolic MCA branch ischemic territorial infarction on the right (*arrows*). The signal intensity is low and similar to that of CSF

lowing for an improved demarcation of lesions with T2 prolongation [136]. Although they may be helpful for depicting small cortical infarctions [41], FLAIR images are by nature T2-WI and, thus, do not show hyperacute ischemic stroke within the first few hours. Furthermore, they have the disadvantage of being associated with relatively long acquisition times, which however can be reduced by applying Turbo-Spinecho techniques [4].

MR angiography (MRA) is a noninvasive imaging tool to assess the vascular status. While DSA remains the gold standard for vascular imaging, MRA gives results with a comparable sensitivity and good correlation with patterns of infarction [101, 164, 376]. Visibility or non-visibility of M2 branches reliably differentiates MCA stenosis and occlusion [101]. Occlusion of farther distal MCA branches cannot be depicted as also has been shown for infarctions with a diameter less than 2 cm [376]. Furthermore, in incomplete occlusions the stenosis grade is frequently overestimated, which can be overcome by motion artifact suppression techniques (MAST), low band width or Multislab 3D-Time-of-Flight Sequences [85, 359]. Also, the original axial acquisitions rather than the maximum intensity projections (MIP) may aid in the assessment of the vessel status [183]. Contrast-enhanced MRA is another technique that improves vascular MRI [290]. New high frequency coils can assess all cranial vessels down to the aortic arch in one acquisition; the only drawback, at least at present, is a study time of several minutes, although rapid sequences exist that can produce an aortic arch angiography within 1.5 minutes. Contrast-enhanced MRA techniques should not be employed if PWI is to be performed, if the maximal MRI contrast dose (triple standard dose) is not to be exceeded and the patient is compliant enough to follow breathhold orders.

Diffusion-weighted imaging (DWI) allows the in vitro and in vivo measurement of Brownian molecular motion of water, a phenomenon first described in 1965 [327]. The distance that water molecules move in these stochastic motions is in the range of a few μm, which is significantly lower than the spatial resolution of MRI. Therefore, these water movements are not directly but indirectly measured. Between the high frequency pulse and the data acquisition, a bipolar pair of gradient pulses are introduced. The first gradient pulse results in a dephasing of proton spins which is completely reversed by the second gradient pulse, if there were no molecular water movement in between. As there is always, if only minute, molecular movement, there will always be a residual dephasing which leads to a signal loss in DWI. The relative signal loss (S/S_0) increases with increasing movement of the water molecules and is mathematically described as follows:

$$\frac{S}{S_0} = e^{-b \cdot ADC} \tag{1}$$

where b is a sequence-specific variable, the so-called b-value. This parameter defines the degree of motion sensitivity of the respective sequence. It is dependent on the strength of the diffusion gradient (G), the duration of the gradient pulse (δ), the time interval between both gradient pulses (Δ), and the diffusion time.

The apparent diffusion coefficient (ADC) is a tissue-specific variable. This parameter describes the amount of molecular movement of water along the direction of the diffusion gradient. Finally, S_0 is the signal intensity without any diffusion weighting (b = 0) (Fig. 4.3).

Besides of qualitative measurements of diffusion, the ADC can be quantified [329], either pixel- or region of interest (ROI)-wise to generate ADC parameter maps. To define the ADC at least two measurements at different b-values have to be performed. Principally, all MR sequences could have an additional diffusion weighting if bipolar gradient pulses were added. Due to their high signal to noise ratio and low susceptibility for artifacts, SE sequences are generally used for DWI [241]. If long diffusion times are measured, it is recommended to use a stimulated echo sequence and introduce the diffusion gradient before the second and after the third 90°-pulse (between both RF-pulses there is only T1 and no T2 relaxation) to achieve the optimum signal to noise ratio [220]. Both sequences can be combined with high speed data analysis techniques such as Turbo-

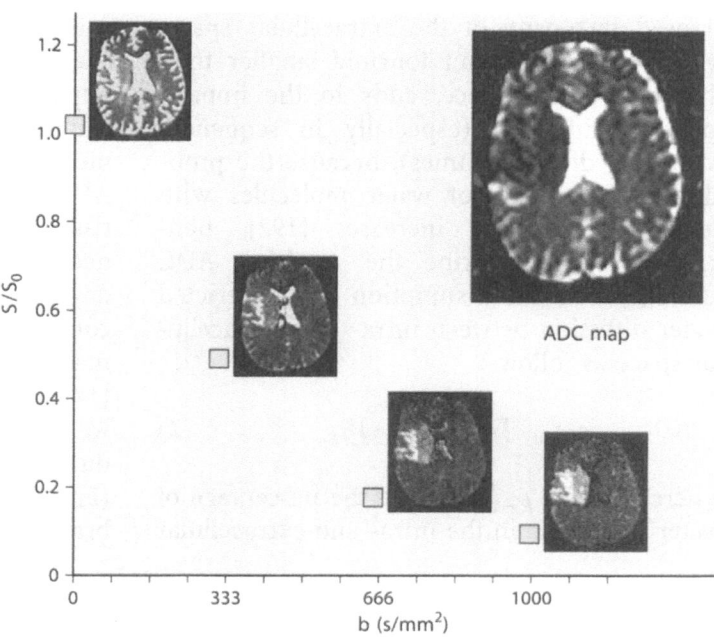

Fig. 4.3. The strength of diffusion-weighting, the ADC map and the meaning of relative signal loss (y-axis) and the b-value (x-axis) are shown. With increasing b-values the motion sensitivity of the respective sequence increases. S_0 is the signal intensity without any diffusion weighting (b=0). What is seen as mild hyperintensity, if at all, on the DWI (b=0) on the upper left becomes with increasing b-values a hyperintense area of 33–50% in the MCA territory including the insular cortex. Infarct is depicted best on the heavily DWI (b=1000). The DWI with different (at least two) b-values are used to calculate the ADC-map, where voxels represent a qualitative measurement of diffusion and low diffusion is hypointense (infarct) and high diffusion is hyperintense (e.g. CSF). To achieve the ADC-value a ROI has to be defined (e.g. a circle put into the infarct) and then the scanner software delivers the mean ADC- (and other) values of this defined area

STEAM, SE-EPI and Stimulated Echo-EPI, which leads to a reduction of motion artifacts and allows the quantification of ADC in the time feasible in the clinical setting [219, 347, 348]. In order to perform DWI with fast imaging techniques, high gradients (>20 mT/m) and ultrashort gradient times (>50 mT/m/ms) are necessary. MR scanners with standard gradient hardware do not allow efficient DWI in clinical practice, a diffusion-weighted CE-FAST-sequence can be used here alternatively. Motion correction can be achieved with navigator-echo sequences. However, quantitative ADC measurements are not possible with this technique as DWI does not only depend on sequence and hardware parameters but also on tissue parameters [53, 146, 221].

Measurement of water diffusion renders pathophysiological tissue information that cannot be obtained with standard MRI-sequences [195, 196]. DWI, earlier than any other imaging modality, allows identification of ischemic tissue changes within minutes after vessel occlusion with a reduction of the ADC [224, 237]. According to animal experiments there is a profound ADC reduction in the infarct core with a less pronounced ADC decrease in the infarct periphery and a good correlation with histopathological findings (40–50% ADC reduction in the infarct core, 10–20% in the infarct periphery [273, 279]). It has not definitively been established, which biophysical mechanisms lead to changes of the ADC; temperature, molecular movement changes and permeability changes of the cell membrane do not suffice to explain the observed findings [26, 75, 353]. The dominating factor for the decrease of the ADC in ischemic brain tissue, however, is probably the shift of extracellular water into the intracellular compartment (cytotoxic edema) with a consecutive reduction of free water diffusion

[238, 287]. It is also considered that the increased tortuosity of the extracellular space, which per se is about fourfold smaller than the intracellular space, adds to the impairment of diffusion (especially in sequences with long diffusion times), because the probability of collision of water molecules with cellular membranes increases [192]. Benveniste et al. describe the resulting ADC (ADC_{res}) with the assumption of unrestricted water diffusion between intra- and extracellular space as follows:

$$ADC_{res} = \rho_{int} \cdot D_{int} + \rho_{ext} \cdot D_{ext} \qquad (2)$$

where ρ_{int} and ρ_{ext} describe the percentage of water molecules in the intra- and extracellular space and D_{int} and D_{int} describe the diffusion coefficient in the intra- and extracellular space [31]. As intracellular water diffusion is impaired by the cell organelles, a net water shift into the intracellular space is accompanied by cell swelling and a decrease of the ADC. With progressive vasogenic edema and tissue necrosis, the initial ADC decrease has a nadir on days 1–2 (animal experiments) or days 3–4 (humans), and thereafter increases continuously, then experiences a pseudonormalization followed by a further increase [179, 207, 215, 384]. In a study in our center we determined the time course of the ADC during the first few days of ischemic stroke (Fig. 4.4) [91]. Eight patients with acute cerebral ischemia were examined by DWI from 2

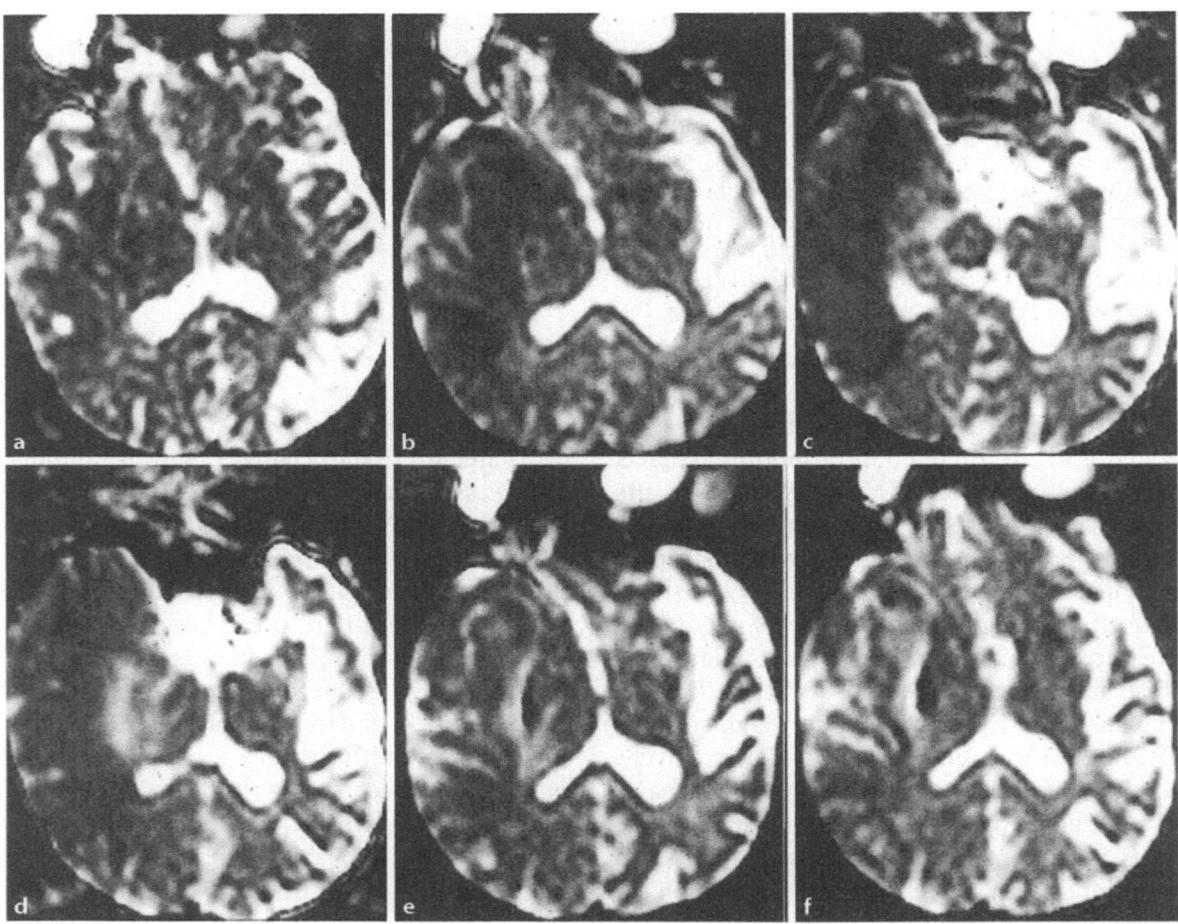

Fig. 4.4. ADC course over time from **a–f** on days 1–3, 5, 8, 10, respectively, after an ischemic infarction of the right temporobasal and insular cortex. Note the profound hypointensity, i.e., loss of diffusion on the first ADC-maps reaching a nadir at day 3; with growing necrotization and vasogenic edema a continuous increase of ADC values to normal values (pseudonormalization) can be observed, which finally result in higher values than at baseline

to 20 h after onset of symptoms. Daily control scans were performed for up to 10 days. ADC values were analyzed from 55 MRI studies. Furthermore, ADC was measured in the tissue that showed a hyperintense signal at the first examination as well as in the contralateral tissue. White and gray matter were analyzed separately. Data were expressed as the ratio of the ADC (rADC) of the lesion to the control region of interest. All patients showed a uniform reduction in rADC from the first hours of stroke to the third day. The rADC increased again from the 4th day up to the point of pseudo-normalization on day 9. The gray matter showed a slightly faster increase than the white matter. Along with T2-WI this allows a differentiation of hyperacute, acute, and chronic stroke. Furthermore, the approximate age of an ischemic stroke can be determined and multiple strokes can be distinguished from a single progressive stroke [91].

On the one hand, DWI has a very high sensitivity for hyperacute ischemic stroke; on the other, it is prone to substantial artifacts that may impair diagnosis. This, however, can at least in part be overcome by the correct choice of imaging technique and sequence parameters.

Motion Artifacts

As DWI measures the movement of water molecules in the scale of micrometers, macroscopic patient motion as well as coherent motion of brain tissue, e.g., the pulsation of the brain, may lead to artifacts, even to global signal loss. The following techniques reduce these artifacts:

- Pulse- or ECG-triggered acquisition: when DWI are acquired at identical points in the pulse cycle, artifacts caused by CSF pulsation or pulsation of large diameter blood vessels can be eliminated [58].
- Navigator-echo-technique: in addition to the acquisition of image data, information about the phase position and spins is obtained. This information is then used to correct for macroscopic lateral or rotational patient movement [77].

- Rapid MR-sequences: by increasing the speed of data acquisition the detrimental effect of macroscopic and pulsatory motion artifacts is substantially reduced. Echo-Planar-Imaging (EPI) sequences, especially when combined with pulse triggering or the navigator-echo-technique, are the optimum choice for DWI, as data acquisition times of less than 200 ms can be realized [210, 323].

Anisotropic Diffusion

When cellular structures have a predominant direction in space such as nerve fibers or tracts, the ADC depends on the direction of the diffusion gradient: while water diffusion is only mildly impaired in the longitudinal direction, water diffusion in a perpendicular direction to the main axis is decreased [24]; this is referred to as anisotropy of water diffusion. In the brain, anisotropy is most pronounced in the white matter, especially in densely packed fiber structures such as the corpus callosum and the corona radiata. For instance, if anisotropic DWI are acquired perpendicular to the axis of such fiber tracts the signal is higher than normal (lower on ADC maps), falsely suggesting a pathological impairment of diffusion.

This effect of anisotropy can be used to obtain information of the regional fascicular or fiber tract anatomy, which may be helpful for neurosurgical procedures; this technique is called diffusion tensor imaging and can also be used to assess myelination and demyelination [242, 254, 266]. The effect, however, is not helpful for the diagnosis of acute stroke as one might falsely diagnose the presence of an ischemic lesion and also under- or overestimate the extent of a true lesion [209]. Anisotropy of DWI (Figs. 4.5 and 4.6) can be eliminated by the following techniques:

- Reconstruction of an isotropic ADC-parameter map: anisotropic DWI are acquired in three different perpendicular diffusion directions (x, y, z axis or read, phase, slice). While this technique allows the reconstruction of an isotropic ADC

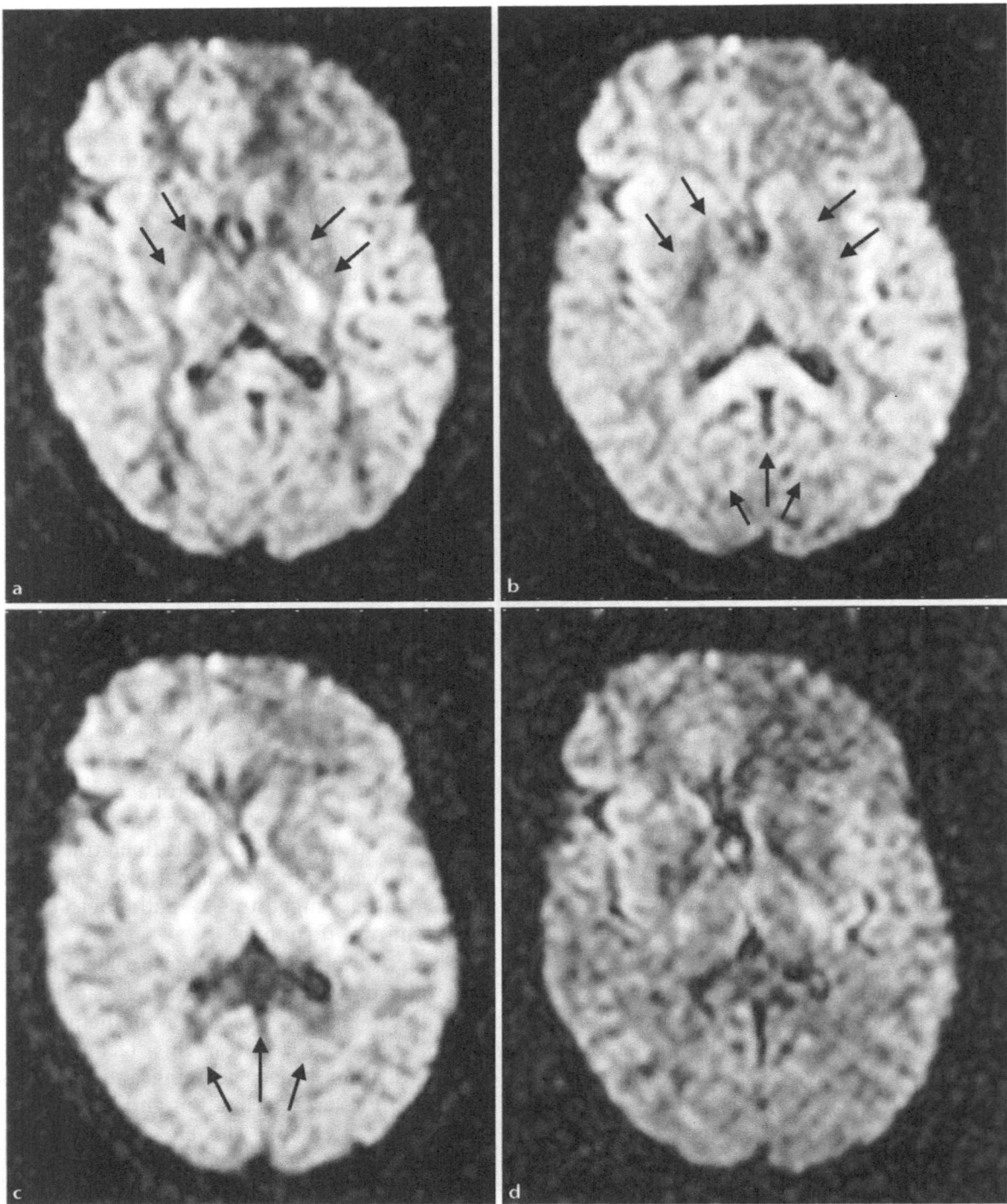

Fig. 4.5. The anisotropy of diffusion is illustrated. **a–c** Diffusion in the three different directions readout, slice, and phase are shown. The arrows depict different diffusion phenomenons in the internal capsule and the posterior commissure. When the DWI slice is obtained perpendicular to the direction of fiber tracts, there is a low diffusion (hyperintense capsule on readout and hyperintense posterior commissure on slice). If obtained parallel to the fiber axis, there is a high diffusion (hypointense internal capsule on slice and hypointense posterior commissure on phase). On isotropic (**d**) DWI, these effects are ameliorated so that pathological diffusion changes are not confused with physiological phenomena of diffusion

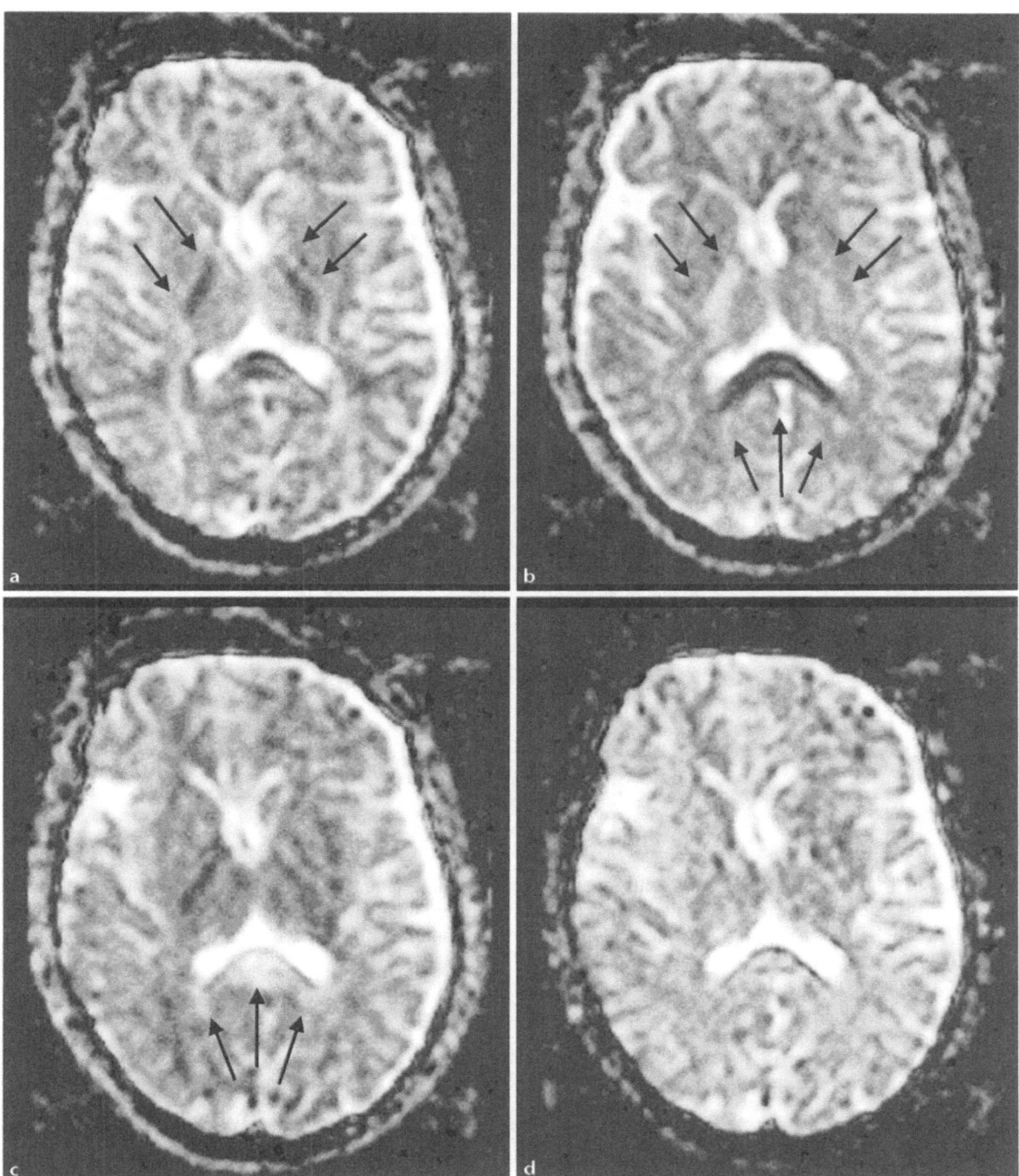

Fig. 4.6. These figures illustrate the anisotropy of diffusion on ADC maps analogous to Fig. 4.5. In **a–c** ADC maps in the three different directions are shown: readout, slice, and phase. There is a low ADC in the hypointense capsule on readout and a hypointense posterior commissure on the slice direction, while there is a high ADC in the hyperintense internal capsule on slice (**b**) and hyperintense posterior commissure on phase direction (**c**). On the isotropic (**d**) ADC map these effects are not present

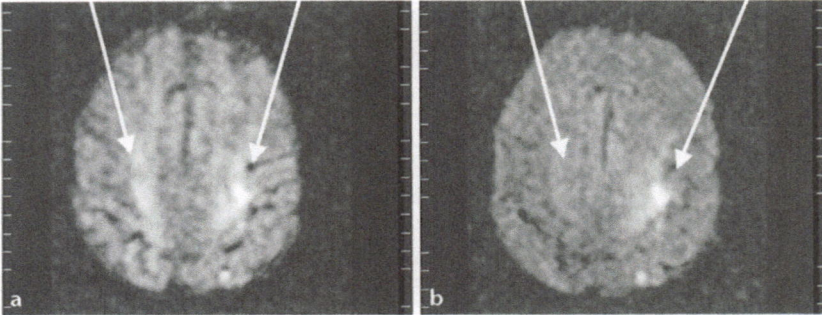

Fig. 4.7. Anisotropic (**a**) and isotropic DWI (**b**). There is a definite lesion in the left parietal lobe of the MCA territory seen on both DWI (arrows). The lesion in the right parietal lobe seen in **a** is physiological diffusion in the corona radiata which cannot be depicted anymore in **b** (arrows)

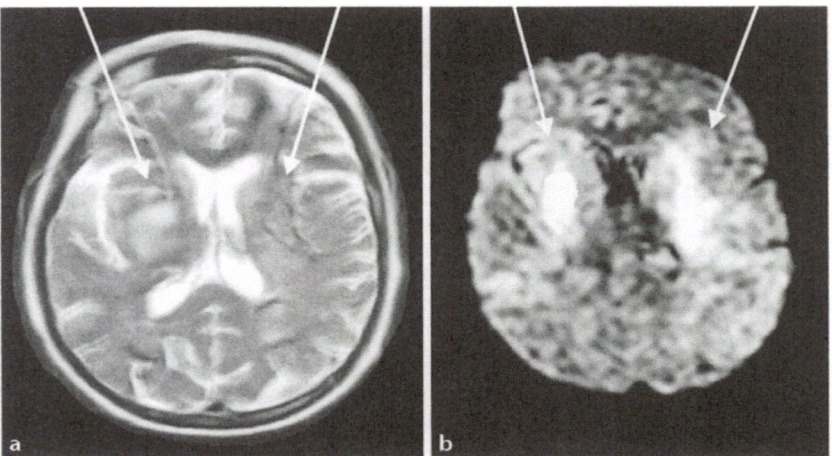

Fig. 4.8. T2-WI (**a**) and DWI (**b**) of a subacute ischemic infarction on the right and a hyperacute ischemic infarction on the left, which is not shown on T2-WI but only on DWI. **b** The DWI shows a strong hyperintensity on the right, which is due to a loss of diffusion *and* a T2-effect of edema as seen in **a** (arrows). The lesion in the left MCA territory, seen only on the DWI (**b**) and not on T2-WI (**a**) is due to diffusion impairment only and depicts a hyperacute ischemic infarction

parameter map, it does not provide an isotropic DW image [266].

Isotropic DWI: a special gradient sequence allows the acquisition of DWI independent of any diffusion direction in one single acquisition [233]. This technique provides isotropic DWI and isotropic ADC-parameter maps. On the other hand, there is no information about anisotropy of diffusion (Fig. 4.7).

■ b-Values

In hyperacute stroke, DWI with high diffusion-weighting are mandatory (minimum b-value 800 s/mm^2) to achieve a sufficiently high diagnostic sensitivity. DWI with standard echo times (80–120 ms) show a maximum signal to noise ratio with b-values of 1100 and 1200 s/mm^2 [269]. Benfield et al., however, showed that lower b-values may also suffice to reliably depict ischemic stroke, as the lesion volume does not change significantly with b-values exceeding 883 s/mm^2 [28]. On the other hand, T2-effects can not be completely eliminated even with b-values of > 1000 s/mm^2 (T2-shine through). DWI alone do not allow the differentiation of hyperacute from chronic ischemic stroke as the first appears hyperintense due to a diffusion reduction (ADC decrease) and the latter hyperintense due to a concomitant T2-effect (Figs. 4.8).

Only when combining DWI with T2-WI (which are negative in hyperacute stroke patients as they show only subacute and chronic lesions) or when using ADC maps can the age of an ischemic infarct be reliably assessed. If low b-values are chosen, the disturbing effects of the high CSF signal and coherent motion should be eliminated [189, 194], so that ADC values can be determined reliably. The error width of the calculated ADC can be reduced when more than two DWI are used [77]. Many centers use two sequences with b-values of 0 and 1000 s/mm^2; at the authors' institution in Heidelberg additional DWI with b-values of 333 and 666 s/mm^2 are used.

In conclusion, animal experiments and clinical studies show that DWI are more sensitive for hyperacute ischemic changes than conventional MRI sequences. However, in order to interpret changes on DWI correctly, a variety of artifacts must be known and identified as such. In the clinical setting of a hyperacute stroke, a lesion on strongly isotropic DWI and a normal T2-WI favor an acute lesion; the maximum information can be obtained, when isotropic ADC-parameter maps are calculated in addition to DWI and T2-WI.

5 Perfusion-weighted MRI (PWI)

P.D. Schellinger, J.B. Fiebach, S. Heiland, K. Sartor

The term perfusion normally refers to the delivery of blood at the capillary level, where the metabolic exchange of nutrients and oxygen takes place. Perfusion-weighted MR imaging (PWI) allows the measurement of capillary perfusion with the dynamic susceptibility contrast-enhanced (DSC) technique. A paramagnetic contrast agent is injected as an intravenous bolus and the signal change is tracked by ultrafast MR sequences in the area of interest [283, 284, 358]. Analogous to concentration time curves obtained with, e.g., Swan Ganz (pulmonary artery) catheters after injection of ice water (temperature probe) or indocyanine green (infrared probe), cerebrovascular (as opposed to cardiac output or vascular resistance measurements) hemodynamic

parameters can be derived from the MR-derived contrast-bolus over time curve. T1-changes caused by the contrast agent do not suffice for PWI as the contrast agent does not permeate the BBB and thus only influences the protons within the capillary vasculature (3–4% of all protons in the brain). A substantially stronger signal change, on the other hand, is obtained by the extra-/intravascular concentration difference, which causes local field gradients that result in a greater shortening of the T2*-relaxation time [97]. The resulting effect has a substantially longer tissue range as compared to the post-contrast T1-WI with the effect that the heavily T2*-WI allow a sufficient measurement of the tissue passage of the contrast bolus (Fig. 5.1).

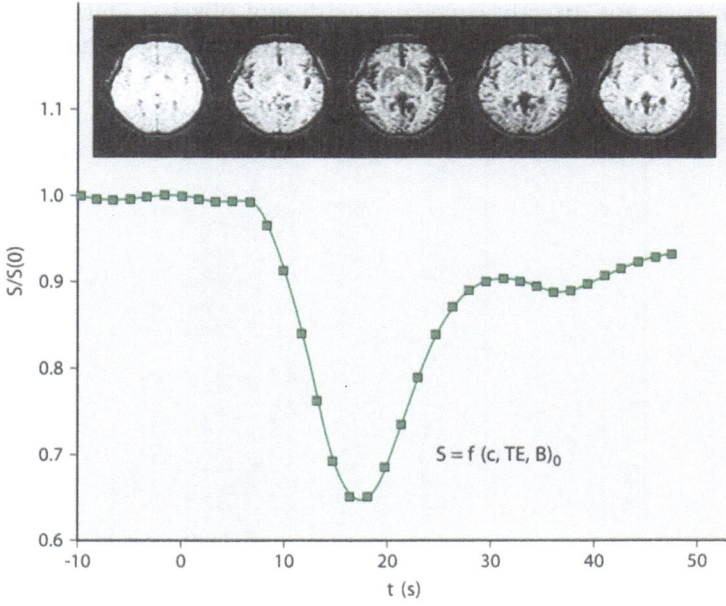

Fig. 5.1. The bolus tracking technique of PWI. Progressing time is shown on the X-axis and concentration of contrast agent as a function of signal strength on T2*-WI is shown on the Y axis. The images above the concentration time curve show that the signal loss parallels the passage of the contrast bolus. This is the unfitted curve. The fitted curve (Fig. 5.5) is created by defining three points on the time axis: baseline, bolus arrival, bolus end

Image acquisition for PWI can be performed with all rapid MR sequences that are strongly T2*-weighted. Frequently used are the following:

■ T2*-weighted FLASH sequences can be used for PWI in MR scanners with standard gradient hardware. Due to the still long image acquisition times only one slice can be assessed per sequence.

■ Gradient-Echo-EPI sequences allow the simultaneous acquisition of several (up to 20) slices (the more slices, the worse the temporal resolution) per sequence. They require, however, special gradient hardware with gradient strengths >20 mT/m and gradient rise times of >50 mT/m/ms). Furthermore, EPI sequences are more prone to artifacts than FLASH sequences.

The contrast bolus passage causes a signal loss that increases with the perfused cerebral blood volume (CBV). In ischemic brain tissue with reduced perfusion or zero perfusion, less (or no) contrast agent is present and T2*-WI remain hyperintense or maintain their high signal [185, 291]. Although the dynamic signal course provides information about the cerebral microcirculation, the relative signal loss is not directly correlated with any physiological parameter. To obtain (semi-) quantitative information about the cerebrovascular hemodynamic parameters, the signal-time curve is used to determine the contrast agent concentration-time curve. This is calculated by the following relation:

$$C(t) \propto \ln \frac{S(t)}{S_0} \tag{3}$$

where $C(t)$ is the concentration of the contrast agent in the brain tissue, $S(t)$ is the signal intensity and S_0 the mean signal intensity before arrival of the contrast bolus. This relation was deduced from numeric simulations [97] and verified through in vivo measurements [284].

The calculation of cerebrovascular parameters is performed exclusively from the first pass of the contrast agent. To exclude recirculation effects, a model function is fitted to the measured values [283]:

$$C_\Gamma(t) = \begin{cases} A\,B^{(t-t_0)}\,e^{-D(t-t_0)}, & t \geq t_0 \\ 0 & , \quad t < t_0 \end{cases} \tag{4}$$

The parameters A, B, D and t_0 are determined by a nonlinear least squares fit. While A, B and D are purely phenomenological parameters, t_0 has a physiological correlate, i.e., the time to arrival of the contrast agent bolus.

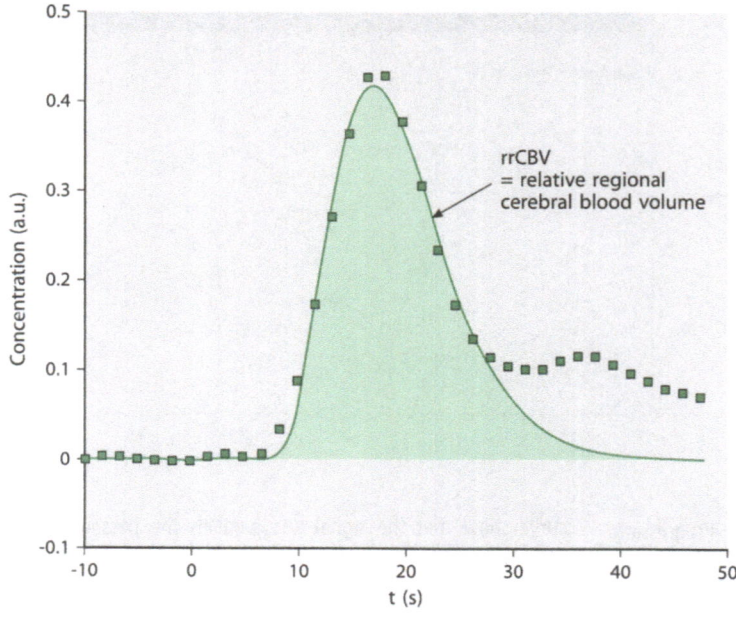

Fig. 5.2. The fitted concentration-time curve is to illustrate what parts of the bolus time curve represent which hemodynamic parameter. Relative regional CBV is calculated as the area under the curve

The fitted model function, aside from the calculation of t_0, also allows the calculation of other important physiological and pathophysiological parameters. With the indicator dilution theory [13, 283, 396], the formula to calculate the relative regional CBV (rrCBV) is as follows (Fig. 5.2):

$$rrCBV = \int_0^\infty C_\Gamma(t)dt \qquad (5)$$

Calculation of the normalized first moment of the concentration-time curve renders the relative mean transit time (rMTT), which is that point in time that divides the area under the curve into equally large areas (Fig. 5.3):

$$rMTT = \frac{\int_0^\infty t \cdot C_\Gamma(t)dt}{\int_0^\infty C_\Gamma(t)dt} \qquad (6)$$

In some centers, instead of the MTT, phenomenological (summary) parameters such as the time from bolus injection to bolus maximum, i.e., time to peak (TTP) or maximum of signal loss, are used. These parameters have the disadvantage that they do not have a direct physiological correlate, are influenced by multiple physiological parameters and without a fitted model function can only be assessed with wide error margins [383]. Perthen et al. have shown with numerical simulations that none of these summary parameters represent a robust measure of perfusion [263]. While formally, rrCBF is equal to rrCBV/rMTT, without measurement of the arterial input function of the contrast bolus an absolute quantification of CBV, MTT and CBF is not possible. Rempp et al. developed a method, where the input function is acquired on a separate MR-slice at the level of a major artery [275]. With a rather demanding and time-consuming postprocessing, the hemodynamic parameters can be quantified albeit with a systematic overestimation of CBV and CBF as compared to PET [385]. The parameters rrCBV, rMTT and t_0 allow a semiquantitative assessment of cerebrovascular changes in ischemic brain tissue compared to the contralateral healthy hemisphere. Calculation of rrCBF from MR data is, in contrast to the model with an ideal bolus [13], not possible [383]. rMTT, however, provides a relative assessment of CBF changes when compared to the healthy side [383]. T_0 does not give any

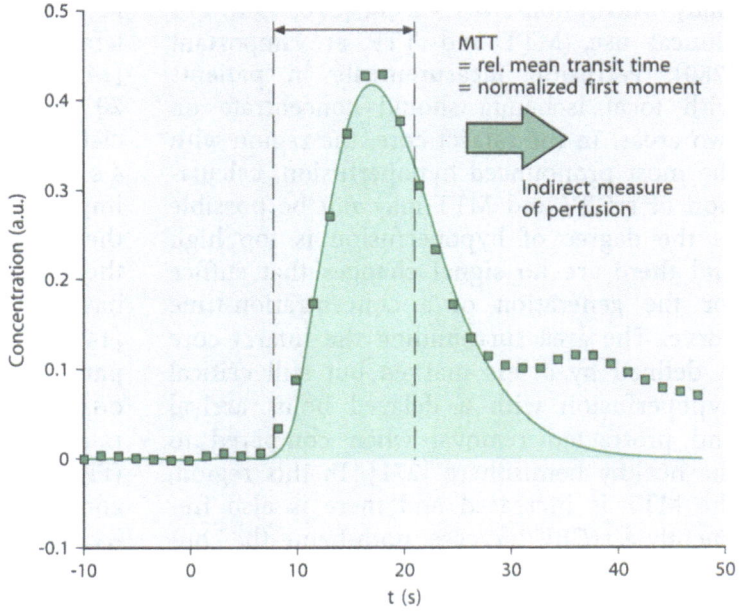

Fig. 5.3. The relative MTT is calculated via the normalized first moment, i.e., that point of time on the X-axis, where 50% of the area under the curve (rrCBV) have passed. This is not the same as the time to peak (TTP). MTT and TTP are identical only when the curve is symmetrical and not skewed. The rMTT is an indirect measure of perfusion

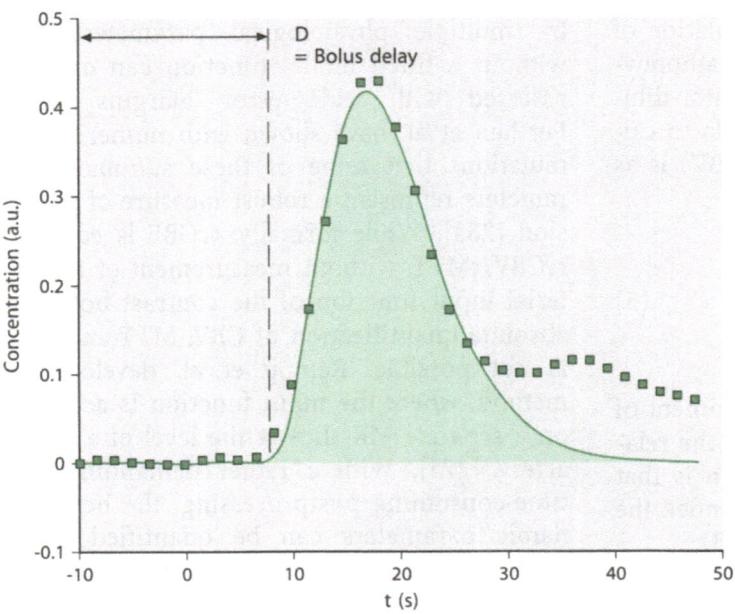

Fig. 5.4. Bolus delay is the time interval D from bolus application to bolus arrival as illustrated on the curve. For instance, in cardiac disease with low output syndromes, the delay may increase and the bolus may disperse

information about the regional perfusion status but about major vessels such as the carotid artery [274]. Animal experiments have shown that the CBV is reduced after vessel occlusion and in early reperfusion increases again to values exceeding the baseline value [140]. Studies in humans, however, demonstrated that rrCBV is an unreliable parameter for the detection of ischemic lesions especially with lesion sizes <2 cm [376, 390]. For clinical use, MTT and TTP are important [280]. Perfusion measurements in patients with focal ischemia should concentrate on two areas. In the infarct core, the region with the most pronounced hypoperfusion, calculation of rrCBV and MTT may not be possible as the degree of hypoperfusion is too high and there are no signal changes that suffice for the generation of a concentration-time curve. The area surrounding the infarct core is defined by a less marked but still critical hypoperfusion with a delayed bolus arrival and protracted removal when compared to the healthy hemisphere [271]. In this region, the MTT is increased and there is also frequently a rrCBV increase, both being the consequence of a reduced perfusion pressure followed by compensatory vasodilation [346]. According to animal studies, the degree of changes on PWI correlates with the ischemic cell damage, the ADC decrease correlates with

the maximum concentration of contrast agent during the bolus passage, and the perfusion deficit during occlusion correlates with the number of apoptotic cells [265, 356]. It is not yet clear which PWI parameter gives the optimum approximation to critical hypoperfusion and allows the differentiation of the infarct core from penumbra and penumbra from oligemia. Most authors, however, agree that MTT (or TTP with the aforementioned problems) give the best prognostic information [14, 15, 302, 373]. One group determined in 20 patients that TTP delays of >6 s are associated with infarct growth and TTP delays of 4 s seem to be the threshold for functional impairment [244]. Another study showed that the amount of infarct growth is predicted by the extent of MTT changes in patients who have not or have unsuccessfully been treated [14]. A recent study by Yamada et al. compared seven different PWI calculation methods and their predictive value (first moment, ratio of area to peak, TTP, rTTP, arrival time (Fig. 5.4), full-width at half-maximum and deconvolution methods) [390]. A high sensitivity that remained robust in patients with underlying vasculopathy, such as carotid artery stenosis, was achieved only with first moment (MTT) and deconvolution methods (Figs. 5.5–5.7).

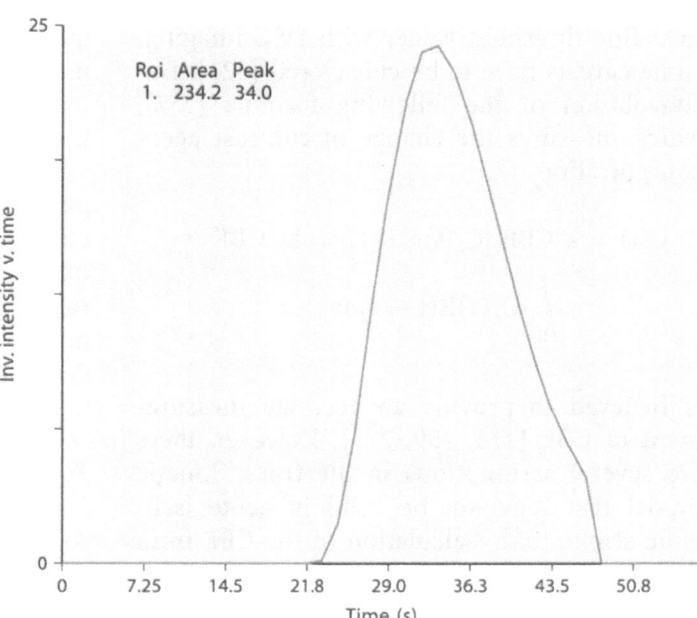

Fig. 5.5. Original image of a fitted curve depicting the contrast bolus passage

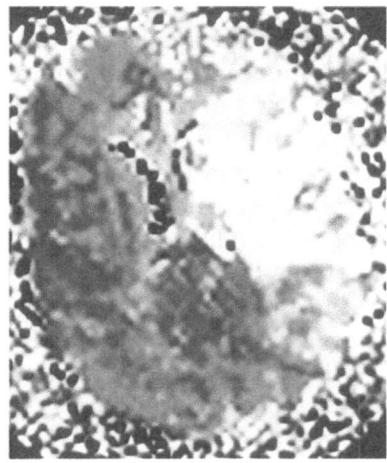

Fig. 5.6. The typical image of a rMTT map is shown. There is a large area of hypoperfusion seen as a hyperintensity when compared to the normally perfused tissue on the right hemisphere. The ischemic area corresponds to the complete MCA territory; hypoperfusion is most profound in the white matter, while less profound in the frontoparietal cortex probably due to some collateral flow via leptomeningeal vessels. This area of hypoperfusion corresponds with a vessel occlusion of the proximal left MCA (M1). Please mind that from PWI alone it cannot be determined which areas are only hypoperfused but alive (penumbra, oligemia) and which are irreversibly ischemic (core)

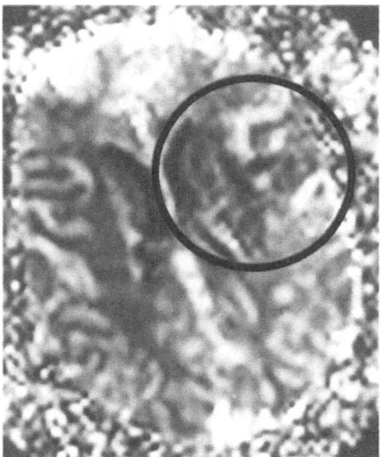

Fig. 5.7. A rrCBV map is shown. As opposed to the readily identifiable hyperintensity on the rMTT map of the same patient (Fig. 5.6), here the hypointensity that reflects vasodilation in the area of hypoperfusion is much more difficult to detect (*circle*). This may be partly improved by software settings; however, the rMTT renders the most reliable estimation of perfusion (see text)

With regard to PWI quantification in order to define threshold values with DSC imaging, some caveats have to be considered [321]. Deconvolution of the following formula [257], which measures the change of contrast agent concentration

$$C(t) = k \cdot CBF \cdot [C_a(t) \otimes R(t)] = k \cdot CBF$$
$$\cdot \int_0^t C_a(\tau) R(t - \tau) d\tau \qquad (7)$$

is believed to provide an accurate measurement of CBF [114, 209, 275]. However, there are several assumptions in the tracer kinetic model that may not be valid in acute ischemic stroke [55]. Calculation of the CBF from Eq. (7) requires knowledge of the arterial input function, which in clinical practice is estimated from a major artery such as the MCA or ICA. However, any delay or dispersion of the bolus from this site to the origin of the capillary bed of the tissue under investigation will introduce an error in the quantification process [54]. Delays of 1–2 seconds (similar to the time resolution used in DSC MRI studies) introduce a 40% underestimation of CBF and 60% overestimation of MTT. These delays are not uncommon in cerebrovascular patients and the errors are further increased with bolus dispersion. Correction for these effects would require modeling of the vascular bed, which is not feasible. A further problem is where to measure the arterial input function. Errors from partial volume effects suggest that a large artery may be optimal, while bolus dispersion and delay suggest that measurement as close as possible to the tissue in question may be optimal. Therefore, there is no complete or unique answer to this question. Another not necessarily valid assumption is that the concentration of contrast agent is linearly proportional to the T2* signal change [284] because the respective proportionality constant k depends on tissue parameters [165] and this may vary with pathology. This constant mainly depends on hematocrit (higher in acute stroke, lower in chronic carotid artery stenosis) and tissue density (fairly constant before vasogenic edema develops) in both large vessels and capillaries. A 30% increase (decrease) in hematocrit leads to a 10% underestimation (overestimation) of CBF and also to false measurements of CBV. The same drawbacks of quantitative measurements hold true for DSC CT, i.e., perfusion CT [13].

Likewise as in DWI, image acquisition and postprocessing in PWI has to be performed, considering technical and methodological factors, so that the measured cerebrovascular parameters are reliable for clinical decision making:

■ Contrast Agent Application

An important factor for data quality is the amount of signal loss during the bolus passage through the region of interest [29]. The signal reduction depends on contrast agent concentration in the investigated brain area which again depends on dosage, concentration, and injection rate of the applied contrast agent [145]. For injection an automatic infusion pump should be used to achieve a user-independent and high injection rate of >5 ml/s. The optimal contrast agent dosage also depends on sequence and scanner parameters. In general, it is valid to say that the stronger the field strength of the magnet and the longer the echo-time, the stronger the achieved T2*-effect is, so that PWI with EPI-sequences in a 1.5 T scanner require the normal dosage of 0.1 mmol gadolinium per kg BW, whereas 1.0 T FLASH sequences require 0.3 mmol gadolinium per kg BW [30]. Patients with low cardiac output syndromes, such as heart failure, may have a diagnostically poor concentration-time curve.

■ Temporal Resolution

Another factor that influences the reliability of the measured cerebrovascular parameters is the temporal resolution of image acquisition and bolus tracking during the first pass of the contrast bolus. In a simulation study, Benner et al. found that at least 8 image acquisitions during the first pass of the bolus are necessary to reduce the error margin to less than 10% [29]. An average bolus pass takes 12–20 s; therefore, a minimal temporal resolution of 1.5 s per slice package is required.

Data Postprocessing

Data postprocessing is time consuming (nonlinear fit, numerical integration), but if the model function is not employed, systematic errors such as second pass and reflow effects will render the hemodynamic data useless.

In conclusion, animal experiments and clinical studies show that PWI with dynamic MRI bolus tracking and adequate postprocessing provides valid hemodynamic information in the form of perfusion parameter maps. On the other hand, PWI has to meet the critique that it renders only a qualitative (at best semiquantitative) index of tissue perfusion, whereas other methods such as SPECT and PET, neither of which have become a standard for patient management, offer accurate quantitative regional cerebral blood flow (CBF) measurements [268]. The evaluation of perfusion status and identification of a tissue at risk by Xenon CT, SPECT or PET, however, are not practical for routine use [158]. While it is not clinically feasible yet to obtain quantitative PWI-parameters that differentiate oligemia from relevant hypoperfusion and infarct core, relative MTT (or TTP) parameter maps may be used to guide clinical management in patients with acute ischemic stroke.

6 The Penumbra and the Mismatch Concept

P. D. Schellinger, J. B. Fiebach

The cerebral perfusion pressure (CPP) is the driving force for transcapillary movement of blood, the cerebral blood flow (CBF) and depends on cardiac output, mean arterial blood pressure (MAP), peripheral vascular resistance and intracranial pressure (ICP). As the CBF is equal to the quotient of CPP and vascular resistance, it can be increased by autoregulatory vasodilation [8]. CBF is constant over a wide range of MAP values as cerebral vasodilation or vasoconstriction counter any changes in MAP; this is the so-called Bayliss effect. In ischemic brain, this mechanism is not functional and CBF is directly dependent on MAP. Cerebral ischemia itself is more often focal than global and is most frequently caused by an acute occlusion of intracranial arteries due to an embolism from an extracranial vessel or from the heart. Less commonly, the cause for an ischemic lesion is an extracranial arterial occlusion resulting in a significant reduction of the CBF, sometimes combined with a drop in systemic arterial pressure. Changes in MAP can then influence CBV as CBV increases with vasodilation and vice versa. There are different thresholds of ischemia and at present a three-compartment model is favored (Fig. 6.1) [187].

CBF values are measured in milliliters per 100 gram brain tissue per minute and normally range from 60 to 80 ml/100 g/min. A drop in CBF down to 20–25 ml/100 g/min is not associated with a loss of function. Also, in individual patients the thresholds may vary, if only slightly. A further reduction of CBF to 10–20 ml/100g/min results in a loss of neuronal function but preserved brain structure. This area of brain tissue thus affected is the so-called ischemic penumbra (semi-shadow, twilight zone) [108, 273]. If CBF is restored in time, the ischemic damage in the penumbra is reversible, and in most instances there is no manifest ischemic stroke on follow-up imaging studies. However, the concept of the ischemic penumbra is a dynamic one that depends on several cofactors such as oxygenation, blood glucose, sufficient MAP and thus CPP, and site of vessel occlusion and collateral status, as well as on duration of ischemia [130]. Sufficient collateral circulation seems to be the most important factor. Large artery-to-artery anastomoses through the circle of Willis, the external to internal carotid distributions (via the ophthalmic artery) and primarily the leptomeningeal collaterals offer relative protection and blood supply to the affected tissue. While in selected cases, large areas of the brain may be permanently supplied by these collaterals only, in most patients the absence or secondary failure of

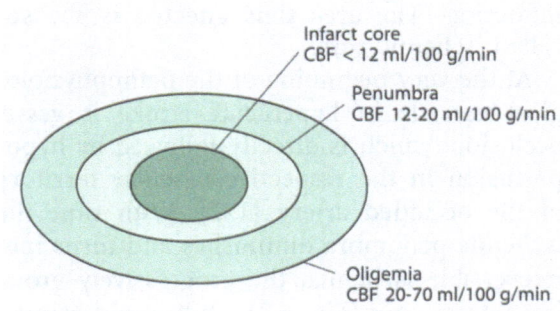

Fig. 6.1. Schematic drawing of the three-compartment model of ischemia. The infarct core with a CBF of less than 12 ml/100 g/min is surrounded by a critical hypoperfusion of 12–20 ml/100 g/min (ischemic penumbra). While the infarct core is irreversibly damaged, the ischemic penumbra has a perfusion that suffices at least over some time to warrant cell metabolism without functional metabolism. If no effective therapy is employed and reperfusion of the penumbra does not take place, this area will turn into irreversible ischemic infarct. There is an outer zone of oligemia that is not critically hypoperfused. This area most likely will survive even if reperfusion does not take place

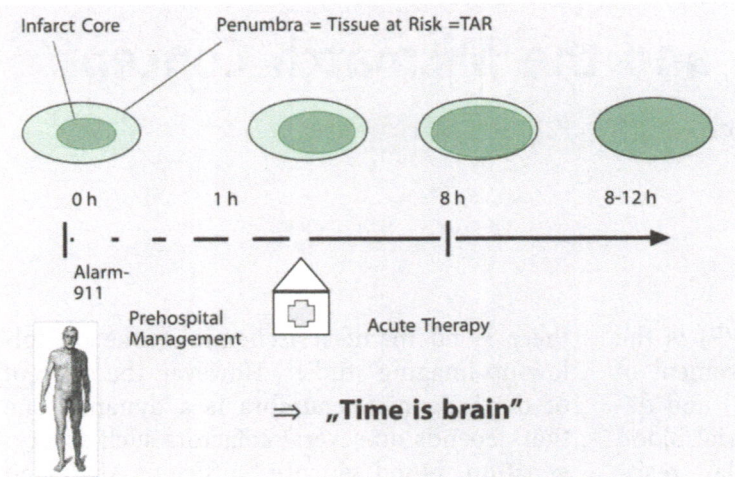

Fig. 6.2. Illustration of the course of the penumbra over time. With progressive time during the first few hours of stroke, the infarct core grows while the ischemic penumbra, i.e., still viable and therefore salvageable brain tissue, shrinks. The earlier the patient is effectively treated, the better the expected outcome. Wasting time in the preclinical and the clinical phase of emergency treatment of stroke reduces the chance for an effective salvage of tissue at risk of irreversible infarction (courtesy of T. Steiner, MD, Dept. of Neurology, University of Heidelberg, Germany)

these collaterals leads to irreversible tissue damage. This variability of the collateral status in each individual results in different morphological and clinical outcomes even in patients with the same site of occlusion. A prolonged hypoperfusion of 15 ml/100 g/min, although primarily in the penumbra range, may therefore lead to irreversible ischemic stroke. Below a threshold of 10–12 ml/100 g/min absolute ischemia is present, which immediately after onset leads to loss of neuronal function and within minutes to neuronal structural damage with irreversible ischemic infarction. The area thus affected is the so-called ischemic core.

At the very beginning of the pathophysiological cascade in hyperacute stroke is vessel occlusion, which is directly followed by hypoperfusion in the respective vascular territory of the occluded artery [127]. With time the ischemic penumbra diminishes and turns into irreversible ischemia, the progressively growing infarct core (Fig. 6.2). Only rapid reinstitution of blood flow within the first hours may disrupt this vicious circle. Although persistent penumbral tissue has been described beyond this time frame, this is more an exception rather than the rule. On the other hand, in individual patients with good collaterals even a later restitution of blood flow may still be beneficial for the patient [32, 362]. It has not yet been firmly established at what point in time reperfusion is definitely ineffective because no viable penumbra is left

or the risk of reperfusion injury exceeds the potential benefit of recanalization [65]. A large combined analysis of six rt-PA trials suggest that after 270 min no significant effect can be expected [46].

The target for most therapeutic interventions for focal ischemia should be ischemic tissue that can respond to treatment and is not irreversibly injured. Such tissue will be defined as potentially salvageable ischemic tissue or tissue at risk of irreversible infarction and must be distinguished from non-salvageable ischemia that has reached a status in which recovery is no longer possible. The attempt to differentiate these two by imaging techniques was made possible by introducing DWI and PWI into the clinical setting. In a simplified approach it has been hypothesized that DWI more or less reflects the irreversibly damaged infarct core and PWI the complete area of hypoperfusion [159, 213]. The volume difference between these two also termed PWI/DWI-mismatch, i.e., PWI minus DWI-volume, therefore would be a measure of the tissue at risk of infarction or the stroke MRI correlate of the ischemic penumbra. On the other hand, if there is no difference in PWI and DWI volumes or even a negative difference (PWI<DWI), this is termed a PWI/DWI-match, according to the model this is equivalent to a patient who does not have penumbral tissue because of normalization of prior hypoperfusion or completion of infarction and total loss of the penumbra (Fig. 6.3) [302].

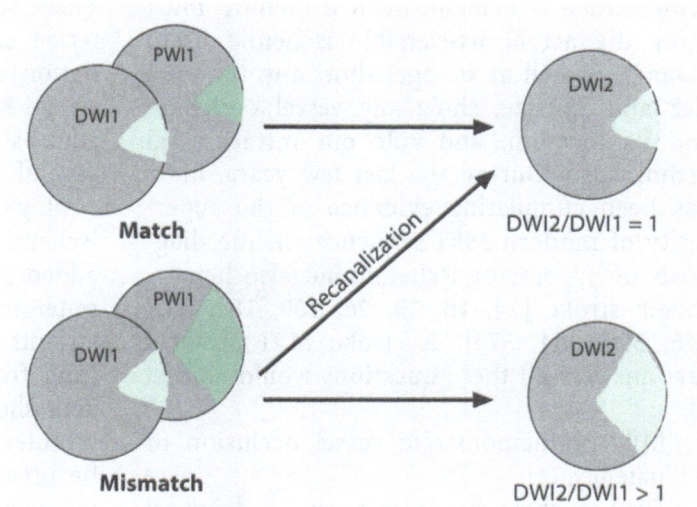

Fig. 6.3. The mismatch concept on PWI and DWI is as follows: essentially there are two types of PWI/DWI constellations that are seen in the first few hours after ischemic stroke. In the first case (upper row), both lesions are of the same size (or PWI is smaller than DWI signaling non-nutritional reperfusion), i.e., a PWI/DWI-match. There is no tissue at risk (the stroke MRI correlate of the ischemic penumbra) and the patient will not experience infarct growth whether thrombolysis is performed or not. In the second case (lower row), the patient has a PWI/DWI-mismatch, which can go two ways. Either he experiences early recanalization which will likely result in a small final infarct (upper row to the right) and a good clinical outcome or he will have a persistent occlusion or too late recanalization which will result in a large infarct with a poor clinical outcome

It may be criticized that this model does not take into account that the PWI lesion also assesses areas of oligemia which are not in danger and that DWI abnormalities do not necessarily turn into infarction [173, 267, 268, 397]. Overall and besides these exceptions, however, this simple model of PWI/DWI-mismatch holds true in most acute patients and stroke MRI findings are consistent with our pathophysiological understanding [302]. It is hoped that by using the mismatch concept patients can be categorized into two groups: those that may profit from a specific therapy to salvage the penumbra and those where no ischemic tissue at risk is present anymore. Furthermore, the patient's individual time window due to his or her individual vascular and hemodynamic situation can be taken into account for decision making.

In summary, the pathophysiological concept of three different zones of hypoperfusion, especially the penumbra concept, may be transferred to imaging findings in stroke MRI. This led to the stroke MRI construct of the PWI/DWI-mismatch, which may be the correlate of the ischemic penumbra and therefore identify the patients who might be effectively treated.

The ideal stroke imaging tool is characterized by several logistic as well as diagnostic aspects. First, the imaging modality in question should be available around the clock at all times including the weekends, which requires sufficient personnel. The method must also be safe for severely ill patients and thus allow monitoring. The time loss for imaging must not exceed 15 to 20 minutes as in hyperacute stroke "time is brain" and each minute lost until an effective therapy is instituted means a loss of penumbral tissue. The ideal stroke imaging tool should provide all the information that is needed to optimally treat the stroke patient. Thus, it does not make sense to primarily choose an imaging modality that cannot deliver all the information that is needed, such as Doppler ultrasound, which may show whether there is a vessel occlusion but does not reliably depict infarct or hemorrhage.

The need for a comprehensive diagnostic tool that allows the identification of all important pathophysiologic aspects of hyperacute stroke is evident. Such a method must show the actual irreversible ischemic brain damage as well as its age, show any tissue at risk and its size, show any vessel occlusion and its location, and rule out intracerebral hemorrhage. During the last few years, there has been cumulating evidence of the superiority of modern MRI sequences in the diagnosis of hyperacute ischemic but also hemorrhagic stroke [14, 18, 23, 26, 160, 184, 223, 226, 306, 344, 373]. A stroke MRI protocol that answers all these questions would consist of:

- MRA to demonstrate vessel occlusion or patency,
  DWI to show the infarct core and infarct age (ADC maps),
- T2-WI to give a more anatomical image of the brain in stroke patients, depict microangiopathic changes, edema, old infarcts, other pathology, etc.,
- PWI to show the complete area of hypoperfusion and derive the tissue at risk by comparing the results with the findings on DWI, and
- T2*-WI (source images from PWI) to show the presence or absence of intracranial hemorrhage.

These sequences suffice to completely characterize each individual stroke patient. As an option or depending on the findings of the stroke MRI protocol, a FLAIR, pre- and post-contrast T1-WI can be added, if needed in several planes. If it is determined that the etiology of the stroke-like symptoms is not an ischemic stroke, other sequences can be added to the protocol as needed. It should be reiterated that, because of the time constraints imposed by the narrow therapeutic time frame, the imaging protocol should be kept short [126]. At present a time loss of 10 minutes when compared to a CT protocol will be offset by the immense gain in additional information.

In analogy, a stroke CT protocol could consist of non-contrast CT to exclude ICH, CTA to assess the vessel status and perfusion CT to show the area of complete hypoperfusion. Unfortunately CT and its dynamic variants are not sensitive enough to reliably depict the infarct core and therefore can not demonstrate the tissue at risk. The reason for this is that CT depicts only secondary and tertiary phenomena of the pathophysiological cascade of stroke. Other imaging modalities such as DSA, PET, or SPECT do not fulfill the criterion that they be comprehensive.

7 Stroke MRI and Intracranial Hemorrhage

P. D. Schellinger, J. B. Fiebach

Non-traumatic intracranial hemorrhage (ICH) accounts for 10–15% of all strokes but up to 25% of more severe strokes [166, 387]. The etiology of ICH in the vast majority of patients are atherosclerosis and arterial hypertension (63.5%), followed by coagulopathies (15%) and vascular malformations (8.5%), and less frequently amyloid angiopathy, vasculitis, intoxication, cavernoma, or cerebral venous thrombosis [285]. In the hyperacute emergency assessment (<6–12 h), computed tomography is the diagnostic standard and modality of choice to differentiate between hyperacute ICH and ischemic stroke [130, 150, 158]. In general, MRI at this stage is considered to be of little value for the diagnosis of ICH or subarachnoidal hemorrhage (SAH) and many authors claim that the sensitivity of MRI for detecting hyperacute ICH is poor [37, 143, 144, 382]. Throughout this chapter we arbitrarily defined hyperacute (<12 h), acute (12 h to 7 d), subacute (7 d to 3 mo) and chronic (>3 mo) stages. While hyperacute ICH is hyperdense on acute CT scans, there is a loss of density with time, and hematoma degradation and the ICH may appear isodense or hypodense. MRI is far superior to CT in the subacute and chronic stages especially with regard to concomitant or underlying pathology [89]. In a study of 129 patients with ICH, Steinbrich et al. found sensitivities of 46% (MRI) and 93% (CT) in the hyperacute and acute stage but 97% (MRI) and 58% (CT) in the subacute and 93% (MRI) and 17% (CT) in the chronic stage [324]. Also, petechial bleedings, discrete foci of contusion, and evidence of residues from ICH were only demonstrated by MRI. This chapter will cover the MRI signatures of ICH in all stages but will focus on the differential diagnosis in hyperacute stroke patients, where stroke MRI becomes more and more important for guiding therapy in ischemic stroke patients. It will also briefly deal with subarachnoid hemorrhage (SAH) and discuss future prospects such as the detection of perihemorrhagic pathologic processes, which may contribute to the morbidity of ICH.

■ MRI Signatures of Acute, Subacute and Chronic ICH

Gomori and Grossman described already in the mid-1980s the stage-dependent signal intensity of ICH in different MRI sequences in experimental [111] as well as clinical situations [109, 110, 119, 120]. The appearance of ICH depends on several factors, such as the MRI sequence used [256, 382], field strength [43, 306, 398], and the oxygen saturation of hemoglobin and its degradation. Other factors are protein concentration, hydration, form and size of red blood cells, hematocrit, clotting, clot retraction and clot structure [34, 59, 64, 109, 143, 157, 176]. As a hematoma ages, the hemoglobin passes through several forms (oxyhemoglobin, deoxyhemoglobin, and methemoglobin) prior to red cell lysis and breakdown into ferritin and hemosiderin. The T2 relaxation rate varies quadratically with the concentration of deoxyhemoglobin [111]. Acute hematomas are characterized by central hyperintensity on T2-WI, whereas they appear isointense on conventional T1-WI. Methemoglobin formation leads to a T1-shortening and therefore to a centripetal hyperintensity on T1-WI, which is also taking effect on T2-WI causing a hyperintense signal. This may allow the approximate classification of the stage and thus age of the ICH. In late subacute and chronic ICH, a hypointense rim caused by the paramagnetic effect

Table 7.1. Signal characteristics of ICH

	T1-WI	T2-WI	FLAIR	T2*-WI
Hyperacute signal 0–12 h	Isointense core and rim, hypointense edema	Hyperintense core and rim, hyperintense edema	Heterogeneous hyper-intensities and hypo-intensities, hyperintense edema	Ultraearly (< 2 h) target-like appearance, heterogeneous or iso-intense core, hypo-intense rim, later rim and core strongly hypo-intense to signal loss, hyperintense edema
Etiology	Oxyhemoglobin (OxyHb) in the core, deoxyhemoglobin (DeoxyHb) in the rim, vasogenic edema surrounding the ICH			
Time course	Growth of the hypo-intense edema	Edema growth, no or little loss of intensity at the periphery of ICH	Mildly progressive, centripetal loss of intensity, increasing edema	Progressive increase of signal loss from the periphery coreward
Acute signal 12 h–7 days	Initially isointense core and rim, later hyper-intense rim and hypo-intense edema	Hypointense core and initially hyperintense then hypointense rim, hyperintense edema	Hypointense core and rim, hyperintense edema	Signal loss in core and rim, hyperintense edema
Etiology	Deoxyhemoglobin in core and rim, vasogenic edema, after 3–4 days from periphery coreward formation of methemoglobin (MetHb)			
Time Course	Growth of edema, centripetal hyper-intensity due to MetHb	Growth of edema, centrifugal loss of intensity	Persistent signal loss	Persistent signal loss
Subacute signal 7 days–3 months	Hyperintense core and rim, later peripheral iso- to hypointensity	Hyperintense core and rim, blooming (increasing signal loss)	Persistent signal loss, blooming	Persistent signal loss, marked blooming
Etiology	MetHb in core and rim, in further course from peripheral coreward formation of hemosiderine (T1-isointense) and ferritine (T1-hypointense)			
Time course	Centripetal hypo-intensity, shrinking	Increased blooming and shrinking	No change	No change
Chronic signal > 3 months	Hypointense scar	Hypointense scar	Hypointense scar, blooming	Hypointense scar, blooming
Etiology	Hemosiderine and ferritine in macrophages, marked T2*-effect			
Time course	None	None	None	None

of ferritin and hemosiderin demarcates the border zone of the hematoma, which is better seen on T2-WI than on T1-WI. Hyperacute ICH presents as an unspecific hyperintensity on T2-WI and cannot be seen on T1-WI unless there is a substantial mass effect. Excellent overviews about this can be found in Osborn, *Diagnostic Neuroradiology* [256] and Sartor, *Diagnostic and Interventional Neuroradiology* [295]. New sequences which are more susceptible to paramagnetic effects of deoxy-hemoglobin however may detect hyperacute ICH. Due to the complexity of ICH appearance in different sequences at different stages as opposed to CT, there is an considerable amount of uncertainty among clinicians and radiologists as to the role of MRI especially in the evaluation of hyperacute stroke (Table 7.1).

Aside from the differentiation between ischemia and hemorrhage, MRI may provide information with regard to the etiology of

ICH. Basal ganglia hemorrhage in combination with older microbleeds or vascular leukencephalopathy implies a hypertensive etiology of ICH as do lobar hematomas in the elderly [88]. Multiple cortical ICH in the elderly may hint towards an amyloid angiopathy [135]. In young patients, additional information from MRA may detect aneurysms, arteriovenous malformations, vasculitis-like changes, such as multiple intracranial stenoses, or cerebral venous thrombosis and thus may make an invasive conventional angiography unnecessary [159, 289].

MRI in Hyperacute ICH

Hyperacute stroke does not only demand a complete diagnostic workup, with which all the important pathophysiologic aspects of hyperacute ischemic stroke can be investigated but also the differentiation between ischemic stroke and intracranial hemorrhage by the radiologist, which is impossible by clinical means only [129, 130]. The diagnosis of ICH is still a domain of CT rather MRI. The need to perform both CT for exclusion of ICH and stroke MRI to guide therapeutic efforts is time–consuming („time is brain"), medico-economically questionable, and also unpracticable [267, 268]. Therefore, characteristic MRI features of hyperacute ICH especially on newer sequences should be described and utilized. Many authors generally claim that the sensitivity of MRI for detecting hyperacute ICH is poor [37, 144]. The appearance of intracranial hemorrhage at magnetic resonance (MR) imaging depends primarily on the age of the hematoma and the type of MR contrast (i.e., T1 or T2 weighted). Immediately after ICH there are intact red blood cells with intracellular oxyhemoglobin within a protein and fluid-rich serum [324]. Oxyhemoglobin is diamagnetic and does not cause any susceptibility effects [256]. The key substrate for early MRI visualization of hemorrhage is deoxyhemoglobin, a blood degradation product with paramagnetic properties due to unpaired electrons. As long as the deoxyhemoglobin is intracellular (contained within the erythrocytes) during the very first hour after ICH onset, it does not cause rapid dephasing of proton spins in T2-WI or in T2*-WI, and, thus, does in theory not allow for a signal loss within the first 12 hours [217, 324]. However, the paramagnetic deoxyhemoglobin changes the local magnetic field gradient and this leads to a dephasing of stationary or moving protons inside and in the vicinity of the ICH [89]. The short T2 observed when deoxyhemoglobin forms is enhanced on higher-field-strength systems (1.5 Tesla) and on gradient-echo images and is reduced with „fast spin-echo" MR techniques [37].

Gustafsson et al. and Küker et al. investigated hyperacute ICH in animal experiments [123, 137, 186]. Both studies performed MRI directly after ICH and within 6 hours thereafter, in Küker's study up to ten days. Gustafsson et al. induced ICH and SAH via injection of autologous blood in 9 rabbits; MRI were compared to formalin-fixed brain slices. ICH and SAH was identified as an area of hypointensity by GE sequences in all animals, which did not change over time and correlated well with histological findings. Conventional spin-echo (T1, T2, PDI) and FLAIR images showed brain isointense lesions which were more difficult to identify. Küker et al. compared 1.5 (N=27) and 0.5 Tesla (N=10) MRI studies in 25 pigs, in which autologous blood was injected intracerebrally via a burr hole [186]. All animals were imaged with T2*-, T2-, FLAIR- and T1-sequences, initially as well as on days 2, 4 and 10 and the imaging data were compared to histological controls. On SWI, the hematoma was shown in all animals, both at 0.5 and at 1.5 Tesla. The hematoma appeared hypointense in 36 of 37 cases and hyperintense with a hypointense rim in one case. Interestingly, findings in that last case correlate well with the clinical observations of Linfante et al. [204]. SAH and intraventricular hemorrhage was seen best on FLAIR images, but not on conventional SE images. In both studies, venous blood was used which may explain why the hypointensity was that profound that early, as the venous blood already is partially deoxygenated, thus, showing more susceptibility effects early on.

There are only a few publications which report a high diagnostic accuracy of MRI for ICH within a time window of 6 hours or less after symptom onset [84, 204, 261, 306]. Patel et al. were the first to demonstrate early MRI

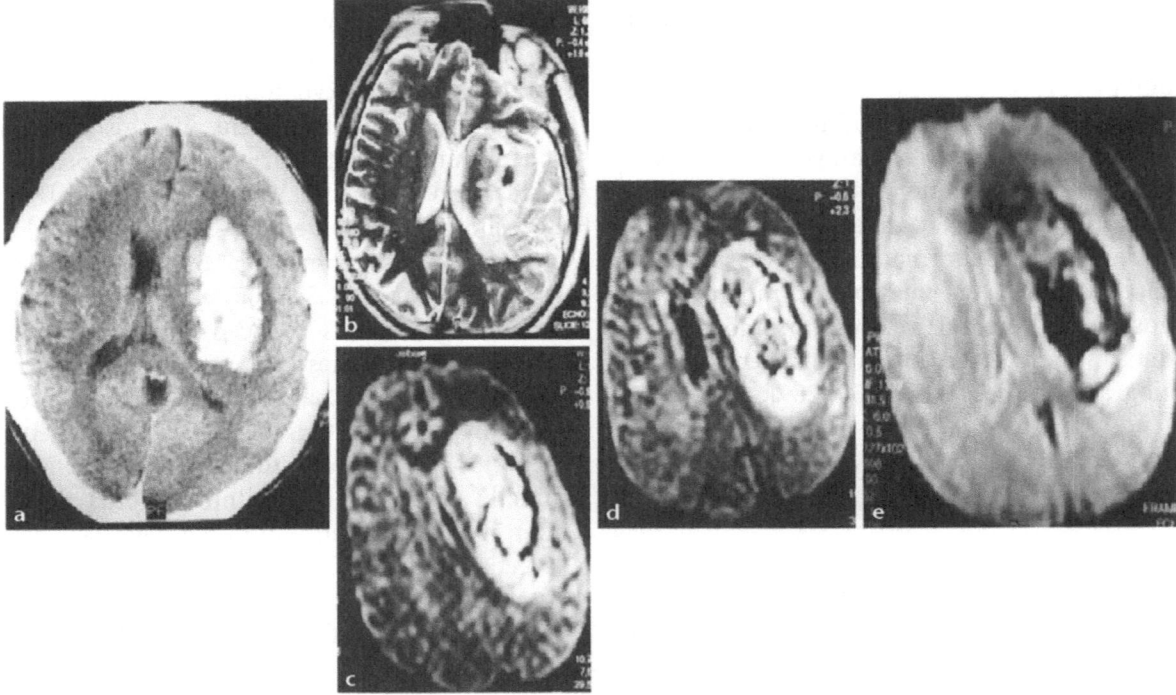

Fig. 7.1. A 40-year-old man with no risk factor other than untreated arterial hypertension suffering from severe headache, plegia of the right arm, grade 3 paresis of the right leg, severe non-fluent aphasia, and forced gaze deviation to the left. CT 2 h and MRI 3 h after symptom onset: The initial CT (**a**) demonstrates a left putaminal ICH and T2-WI (**b**) an irregular hyperintense putaminal lesion on the left. DWI (**c**), FLAIR (**d**), and T2*-weighted PWI (**e**) source images show an increasing area of signal loss within the core of the left-sided hematoma with a heterogeneous appearance caused by small amounts of deoxyhemoglobin

changes in susceptibility-weighted T2*-WI within 5 hours in six patients with acute ICH [261]. Schellinger et al. compared CT and stroke MRI findings in 9 patients with acute ICH in a standardized stroke imaging protocol (CT, DWI, PWI with T2*-W source images, T2-WI, FLAIR images, MRA); all patients received CT and MRI within a 3 to 6 h time window [306]. ICH was unambiguously identified on the basis of all stroke MRI sequences. Volumetric analysis showed a good raw correlation of hematoma volumes in all MRI images compared to CT. As already reported by Rosen et al., images obtained with sequences with a high sensitivity for susceptibility effects (T2*-WI, FLAIR) generally overestimate the actual hematoma size in comparison to the lesion volume assessed on CT [283]. Hematoma volumes on DWI (median and mean difference 3.97%/-4.36%, SD $\sigma=$ 37.42%) followed by FLAIR (median and mean difference -2.91%/-6.25%, SD $\sigma=$ 28.39%) corresponded best with lesion size on CT. Conventional T2-WI substantially underestimated (median and mean difference 17.24%/12.98%, SD $\sigma=34.46\%$) and T2*-WI substantially overestimated (median and mean difference -17.94%/-18.86%, SD $\sigma=-24.45\%$) the hematoma size. The typical appearance of ICH on the MRI images was a heterogeneous focus of high and low signal intensities. With increasing susceptibility weight, the central area of hypointensity became more pronounced. The T2*-WI showed no or few areas of hyperintensity, or merely a faint ring around a central core of signal loss (Figs. 7.1 and 7.2).

Linfante et al. successfully investigated 5 hyperacute ICH-patients with MRI between 23 minutes and 2 hours from symptom onset [204]. They reported a characteristic signal- and evolution pattern of hyperacute ICH, dividing the lesion into three parts. In the very first minutes after symptom onset, the center of the lesion appears heterogeneous on all

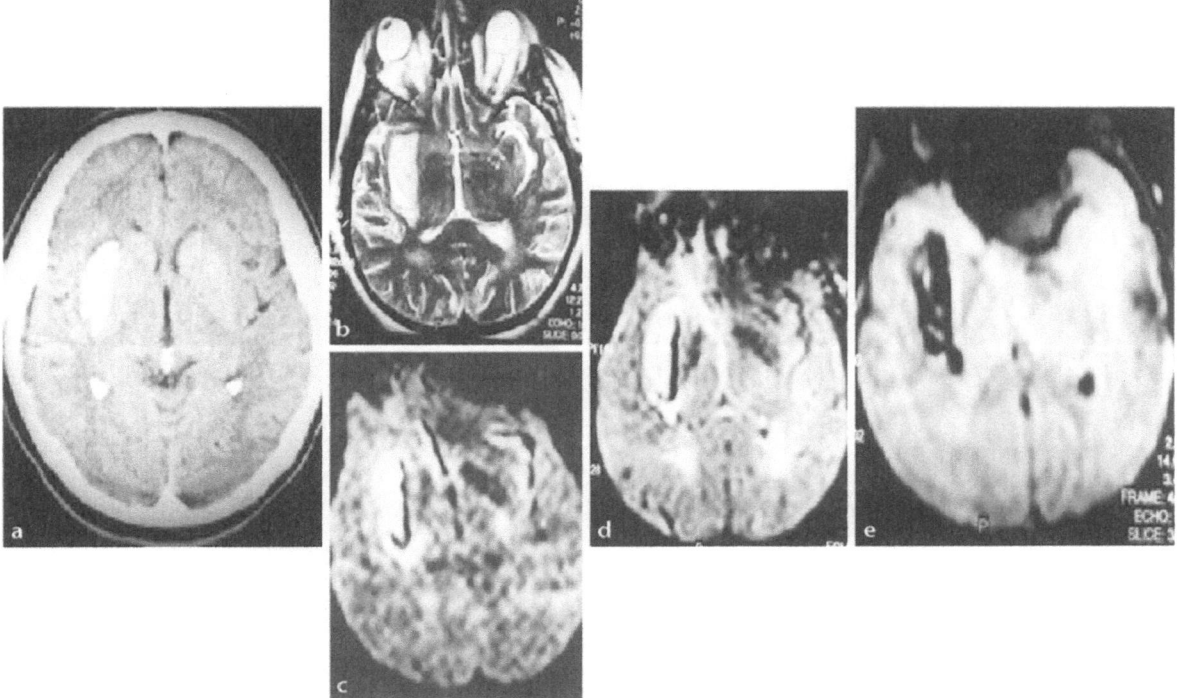

Fig. 7.2. A 65-year-old woman with arterial hypertension and obesity presenting 4 hours after symptom onset with somnolence, grade 2–3 sensorimotor hemiparesis on the left side, incomplete head and eye deviation to the right, moderate dysarthrophonia, and incomplete hemineglect to the left. CT 1 h 30 min and MRI 3 h 45 min after symptom on-

set: (**a**) The initial CT shows an ICH located in the right external capsule, (**b**) T2-WI shows the same lesion as an unspecific hyperintense signal. DWI (**c**) and FLAIR (**d**) revealed an irregular hyperintense putaminal lesion on the right with a hypointense core more prominent on the sequences with a stronger weight on susceptibility effects and strongest on T2*-WI (**e**)

images (T2-WI, T2*-WI, T1-WI), which is due to a local predominance of oxyhemoglobin. The periphery of the hematoma is hypointense on susceptibility-weighted images more than on T2-WI and shows a progressive enlargement over the next minutes and first few hours. This is due to a progressive centripetal increase in concentration of deoxyhemoglobin. There is a surrounding rim, which appears hyperintense on T2-WI and T2*-WI but hypointense on T1-WI and represents perifocal vasogenic edema (Fig. 7.3).

While both authors [204, 306] suggest that stroke MRI is diagnostic in the evaluation of hyperacute ICH, they conclude consistently that the randomized and prospective acquisition of a larger group with blinded evaluation is needed to confirm these preliminary observations. These results support the hypothesis that small amounts of deoxyhemoglobin are present within the very first minutes after onset of ICH and detectable by susceptibility-

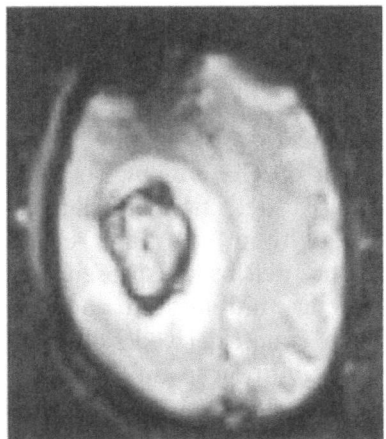

Fig. 7.3. Hyperacute ICH on the right side. T2*-WI 1 h 25 min after symptom onset show the characteristic target-like appearance of ICH with an isointense signal in the core (oxyhemoglobin), a hypointense inner rim (signal loss due to deoxyhemoglobin) and a hyperintense outer rim (T2-effect of vasogenic edema). With elapsing time there will be a centripetal progress of the hypointensity towards the core of the ICH

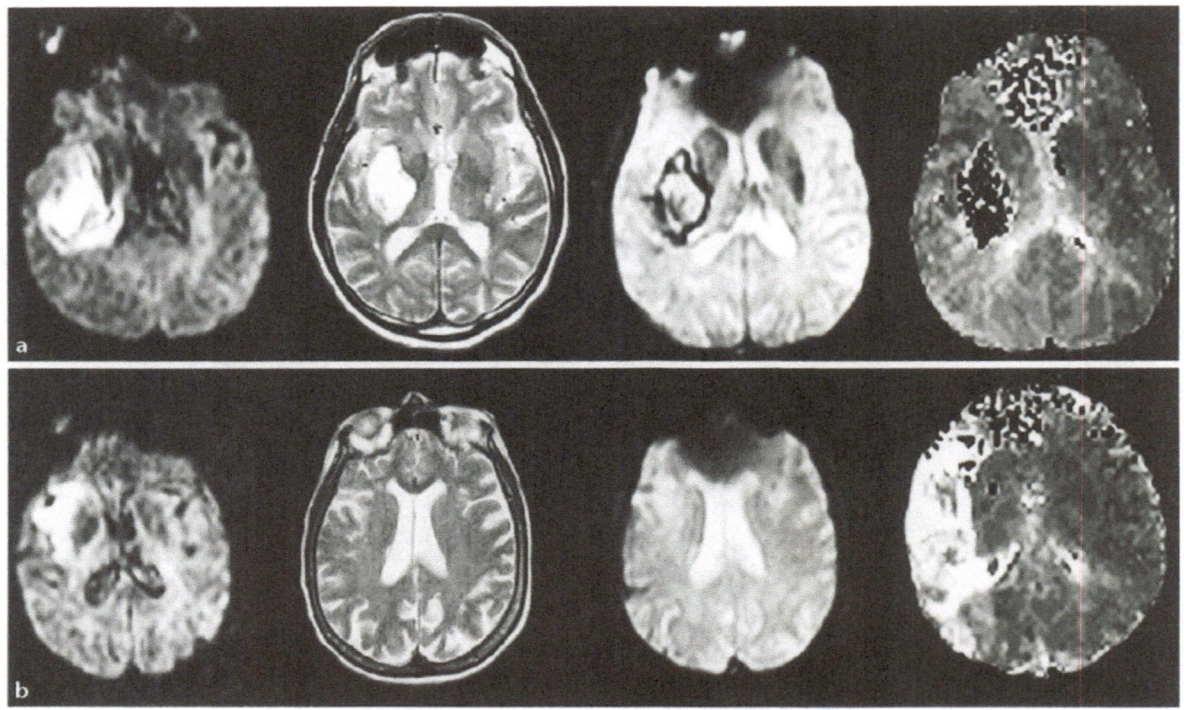

Fig. 7.4. The different appearance of hyperacute ICH and hyperacute ischemic stroke on stroke MRI. (**a**): A 45-year-old patient with a right-sided thalamic bleed of hypertensive etiology 35 min after symptom onset. From left to right DWI show an unspecific hyperintensity (OxyHb) with a small hypointense rim (DeoxyHb) and vasogenic edema (T2-shine through). There is an also unspecific hyperintensity on T2-WI, while the T2*-WI shows the target sign with a heterogeneous mostly isointense core (OxyHb) and the dark rim (DeoxyHb). PWI shows a signal loss and a mild perihemorrhagic hypoperfusion. The MRA (not shown) was normal. (**b**) A 57-year-old patient with an insular MCA infarction on the right side 48 min after symptom onset. Hyperintense lesion that does not look different to that of the ICH on DWI. In contrast, the normal T2-WI and T2*-WI show the characteristic differential features of ICH and ischemic stroke. There is an apparent hypoperfusion of nearly the complete MCA territory sparing the basal ganglia and a large PWI/DWI-mismatch. The MRA (not shown) showed a distal MCA mainstem occlusion corresponding to the area of hypoperfusion

weighted MRI sequences. T2*-WI are suited best for the diagnosis of ICH, which also holds true for the qualitative detection of relatively small hematomas without a mass effect. Further information, such as the presence of space occupying edema, midline shift, and ventricular hemorrhage, is best derived from conventional T2-WI. In addition to the standardized stroke protocol, postcontrast T1-WI scans may be obtained after PWI if another primary disease is suspected (e.g., apoplectic glioma or metastases). Multicenter trials to acquire larger patient numbers have finished recruiting. Preliminary results (ICH and ischemic stroke < 6 h with 63 patients in each group) from blinded reading show a 100% sensitivity and specificity for ICH but interestingly a lower specificity for ischemic stroke (unpublished

data). Figure 7.4 illustrates the difference between ischemic stroke and ICH.

◾ MRI in Subarachnoid Hemorrhage

CT is also the (imaging) standard of care for the diagnosis of SAH [316, 355], with a sensitivity of 85–100%. The CT diagnosis of SAH may be difficult in the posterior fossa due to bone artifacts as well as with small amounts of blood. In the subacute stage, the sensitivity of CT for SAH diminishes substantially with sensitivities of 50% after 1 week, 30% after 2 weeks and ≈0% at 3 weeks [355], necessitating the diagnostic gold standard in SAH, the lumbar puncture. There is currently only scarce information about the sensitivity of stroke MRI for SAH. The first assumptions that MRI may also be suitable in the diagnosis of acute SAH were derived from in vitro studies [56, 218]. In subacute SAH (5 days to 2 weeks), MRI with fluid attenuated inversion recovery (FLAIR) sequences and proton density (PD) weighted images is clearly superior to CT (sensitivity 100% versus 45%) [249]. Some investigators reported that MRI may also be effective in the diagnosis of acute SAH [63, 162, 216, 248, 250]. Conventional T1-WI and T2-WI were shown to be ineffective in the diagnosis of acute SAH with sensitivities of 35–50% [252]. This may in part be due to the fact that the rules, which apply for intracerebral degradation of ICH, may not be valid for SAH due to a higher oxygen partial pressure in cerebrospinal fluid (CSF) [120] and that the formation of blood clots which also causes T2-shortening is impaired [382]. The paramagnetic susceptibility effect, which may be utilized to detect ICH, is not suitable for the detection of SAH as the latter frequently is localized in the vicinity of the cranial vault or skull base, which are areas prone to artifacts. A rise in CSF-protein concentration leads to a T1-shortening and therefore signal intensity increase, which is seen better on PD-WI than T1-WI [162, 297], an observation contradicted by other authors [10, 11]. The detection of SAH may be improved by using PD-WI with shorter repetition times (TR) to visualize the T1-effect [388]. FLAIR sequences have been reported to be suitable for the diagnosis of not only subacute but also acute SAH [218, 247–250]. The latter studies have all been performed with low field scanners (≤0.5 Tesla); however, with increasing field strengths and faster FLAIR sequences (usually 10 to 15 min, TURBO-FLAIR ≈ 3 to 6 min) there also are more pulsation artifacts, which may impair their sensitivity for SAH. Wiesmann et al. recently reported a 100% sensitivity for the combined use of PD-WI and FLAIR images in 19 patients [388]. Artifacts, which were seen in one third of their patients could be determined as such by the combined use of PD-WI and FLAIR images. All PD and FLAIR studies were negative in 10 control patients. Also, newer MRI sequences such as MRA, DWI and PWI may be useful to detect early complica-

tions of SAH such as vasospasm and spreading depression [52]. MRA and DSA provide complementary information with regard to aneurysm detection rather than one method being better than the other [156]; however, when SAH is diagnosed, DSA is still the diagnostic and in certain instances therapeutic method of choice.

In a subset of 5 low grade SAH patients (Hunt and Hess Score I and II), we found a slightly hyperintense signal in all patients on PDI [93]. Compared to CT, the extent of hyperintensity on PD-WI was similar. In four cases a signal hyperintensity was visible on DWI in the subarachnoid space. In two patients the left ambient cistern was hyperintense, similar to the hyperdensity seen on the CT scan. T2*-WI revealed signal changes in four patients, apparent as a hypointense signal located in the CSF space, similar to the hyperintensity seen on DWI. Perfusion maps were completely normal in all patients. The relative MTT was not prolonged nor did the relative rCBV reveal any changes surrounding the affected cisterns in any patient. None of the patients had a symptomatic aneurysm, and MRA demonstrated a contralateral aneurysm in one patient only (Fig. 7.5).

Rordorf et al. reported on multiple infarctions in a cohort of six SAH patients. These patients developed signs of cerebral ischemia due to vasospasm around the eighth day after SAH. In those patients, DWI was performed between 9 and 12 hours after the new onset of symptoms. DWI signal hyperintensities were encircled by a huge malperfused lesion seen on PWI. These lesions occurred in regions supplied by vessels in which spasm had been clearly diagnosed by angiography [282]. The use of DWI in vasospasm was investigated by Condette-Auliac and colleagues in symptomatic and asymptomatic SAH patients [71]. They observed DWI lesions with a decrease in the ADC not only in symptomatic SAH patients but also in seven patients with stable clinical findings. In three of these cases, they observed a transient decrease in ADC. In four patients with normal ultrasound findings, there was no tissue ADC decrease. Normal parenchymal signal on DWI was also observed by Hadeishi and colleagues in 27 patients with low grade SAH [134]. In five patients with grade 4

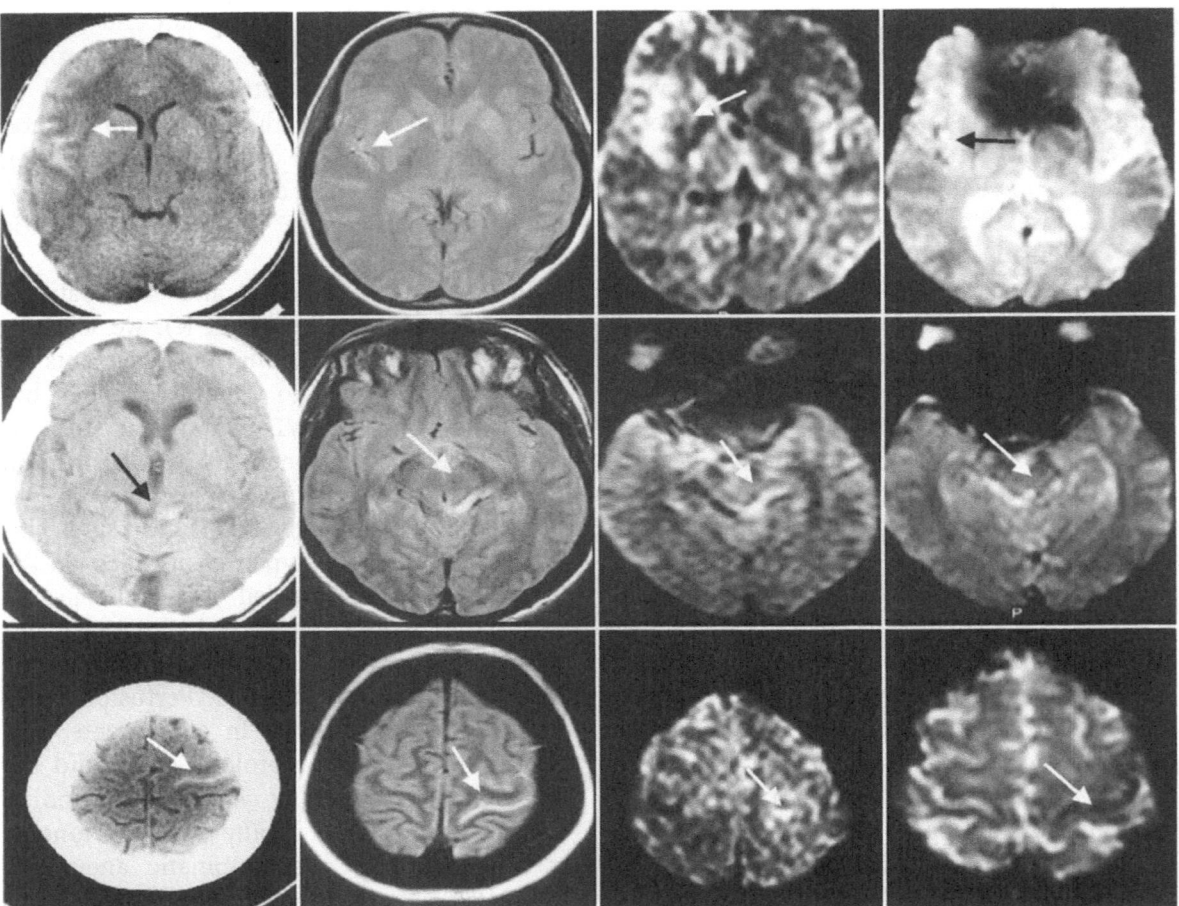

Fig. 7.5. Three patients with SAH Hunt and Hess stage I or II. SAH was visible as a hyperdensity on CT in all patients (1st column). On PD-weighted images (2nd column) the hyperacute hemorrhage appears hyperintense. SAH was hyperintense on DWI (3rd column) in all patients as a result of clot formation with a consecutive decrease of diffusion. On EPI T2*-weighted source images (4th column) there was hypointensity due to signal loss through susceptibility effects at the site of hemorrhage

or 5 SAH, they detected cortical hyperintensities in the supratentorial cortex but normal findings of the basal ganglia and cerebellum. In our cohort of low grade SAH, we did not observe a diffusion decrease in the brain tissue. This is comparable to the findings in Hadeishi's cohort. In contrast to others, we detected diffusion abnormalities in the subarachnoid space exactly where blood was visible on CT. The hyperdensity of SAH on CT is caused by the progress of clot formation that causes a local packed cell volume in the subarachnoid space [116]. This early clot formation may lead to the restricted diffusion that we observed in four of five patients. We suggest that this diffusion decrease localized in the subarachnoid space was caused by a reduced extracellular space. Formation of a fibrin network may also result in a diffusion decrease. Further animal or phantom studies should be conducted to prove this hypothesis. On PWI we did not observe any perfusion abnormality. The perfusion maps seemed to be useless if patients had been designated H&H grade I or II. However, the EPI T2*-weighted source images showed a signal decrease based on a very early susceptibility effect in SAH despite the higher oxygen tension in CSF. Due to the high sensitivity to susceptibility effects, these images may miss signal changes in the CSF at the posterior fossa. The susceptibility caused by the petrous bone makes it impossible to evaluate the peripontine cisterns. Iron in the form of Fe^{3+} and Fe^{2+} is paramagnetic. The minor hemorrhage did not cause any early vasospasm and the absence of a DWI/PWI-mismatch within the first days after ictus and the absence of focal deficits and vasospasm was consistent with the good outcome in all of our patients. Therefore, distinct stroke MRI findings in acute SAH exist that allow the differentiation of SAH from ICH and ischemic stroke. Further studies aimed at the diagnostic reach of stroke MRI in acute SAH are worthwhile.

Future Prospects of Stroke MRI in ICH

There is still controversy with regard to which patients should receive the best medical treatment and whom should receive surgery [169, 230]. In general, patients with mild symptoms and small ICH, severe symptoms and large ICH as well as deep gray matter ICH should not be operated, because surgery does not affect the natural disease course and may even lead to complications and deterioration in patients with mild symptoms or basal ganglionic hemorrhage [90]. Conversely, young patients with a low comorbidity, moderately sized right hemispheric ICH, moderate clinical symptoms at presentation with a rapid deterioration are likely to profit from hematoma evacuation, especially when microsurgical techniques are applied [12]. There are inconsistent data with regard to the pathologic processes in the vicinity of the ICH and their contribution to acute and chronic clinical deficit. Some authors postulate the presence of perihemorrhagic ischemic lesions (animal experimental data) whether caused by toxic effects, apoptosis or reduction of cerebral blood flow [51, 78]; others deny this [240]. In clinical studies evidence has also been provided for [81, 174, 357], and against [152, 393] the presence of ischemic perihemorrhagic areas. Results of the studies by Videen et al. and Zazulia et al., however, suggest that oligemia may be reactive to ICH and represent a reduced metabolic oxygen rate with a constant oxygen extraction fraction rather than being pathologic oligemia or ischemia [357, 393]. Kidwell et al. used a stroke MRI protocol to examine whether there are perihemorrhagic changes on DWI [174]. Twelve patients presenting with hyperacute, primary ICH undergoing CT scanning and diffusion-perfusion MRI within 6 hours of symptom onset were reviewed. They used an automated thresholding technique to identify decreased ADC values in the perihematomal regions. Perfusion maps were examined for regions of relative hypo- or hyperperfusion. The median hematoma volume was 13.3 mL (range 3.0 to 74.8 mL). MRI detected the hematoma in all patients on SWI. In six patients who underwent perfusion imaging, no focal defects were visualized on perfusion maps in tissue adjacent to the hematoma; however, five of six patients demonstrated diffuse ipsilateral hemispheric hypoperfusion. On DWI, perihematomal regions of decreased ADC values were identified in 3 of 12 patients. All three subsequently showed clinical and radiologic deterioration leading to the authors' conclusion that the presence of a rim of decreased ADC outside the hematoma correlates with poor clinical outcome. The role of the diffuse ipsilateral hemispheric hypoperfusion with a lack of a focal zone of perihematomal decreased blood flow in any patient still has to be established. Another small pilot study utilized a stroke MRI protocol with T2-WI, FLAIR, DWI, PWI and MRA to evaluate ICH [303]. There were perihemorrhagic perfusion deficits according to PWI in all 9 patients, and large deficits in 3 of 9 patients, while there were no manifest ischemic infarcts according to DWI. However, whether this was due to the increased intracranial pressure, local compression of the middle cerebral artery, diaschisis, toxic effects of blood products or other mechanisms cannot be answered at this point (Fig. 7.6). Further animal studies and a prospective clinical study, which may shed more light on the pathophysiological, clinical and prognostic relevance of a perihemorrhagic zone of cerebral impairment, are currently underway. Preliminary unpublished data in 32 patients did not show any perihemorrhagic signs of ischemia according to DWI and minor perihemorrhagic hyperfusion, which was not correlated with clinical outcome consistent with the findings of Zazulia et al. [393].

In conclusion, in hyperacute stroke it is of utmost importance that diagnostic efforts be as specific and efficacious as possible, especially with the time constraints imposed by

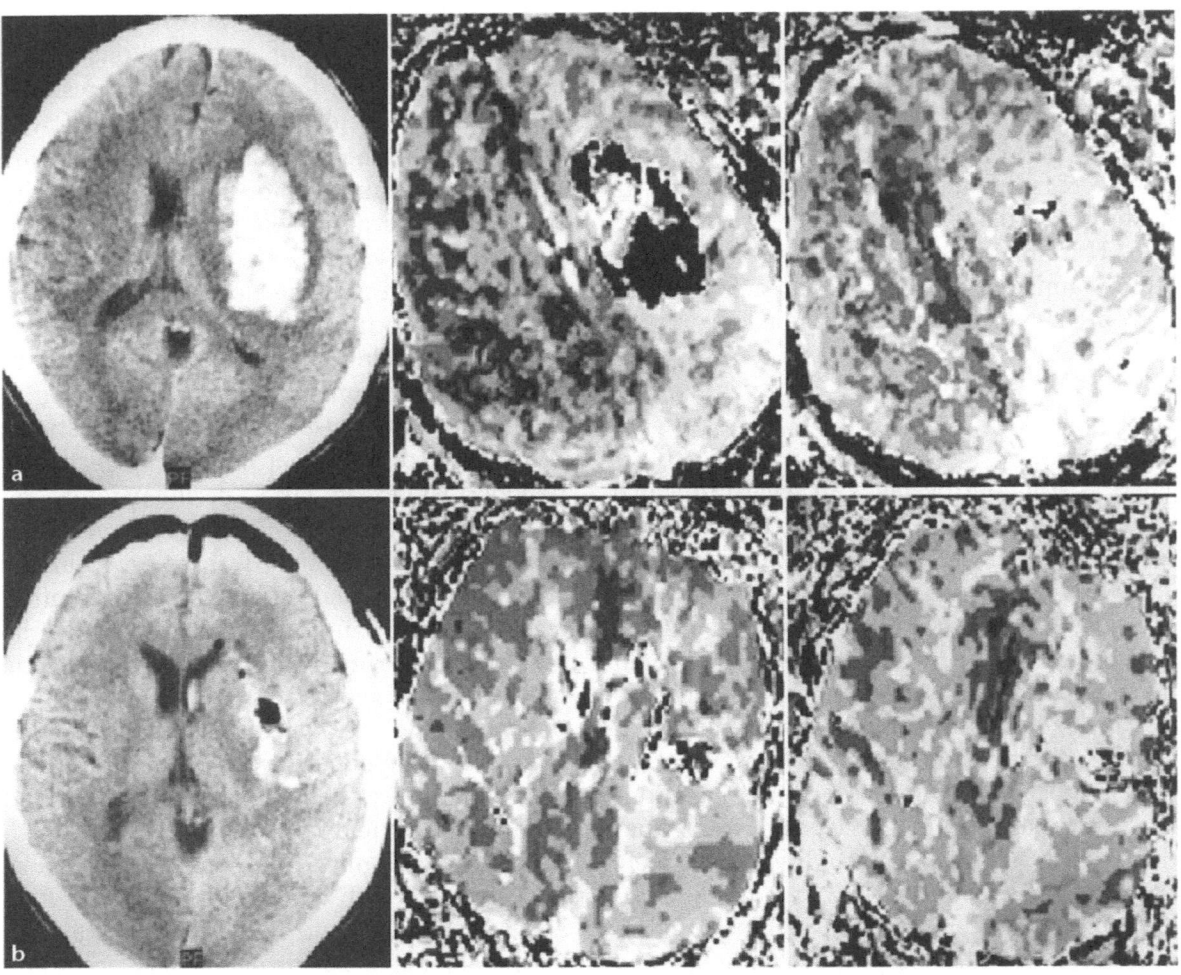

Fig. 7.6. (a) A 41-year-old patient with right-sided hemiplegia and aphasia. Baseline CT shows a large basal ganglia ICH 2 h after symptom onset (*left*). Perfusion-weighted images (PWI, MTT-maps) show a large perfusion deficit (hyperintensity) of the complete left hemisphere (*middle and right*). **(b)** The same patient as upper row 24 h after symptom onset. Surgical removal of the hematoma as seen on the postsurgical CT (*left*). Normalization of perfusion disturbance on the left hemisphere according to PWI (*middle and right*) with small artifacts in the former ICH cavity due to susceptibility (T2*) effects

acute therapies for ischemic stroke such as thrombolytic therapy. Surprisingly, though, MRI is still not generally considered to be the primary and only diagnostic tool in hyperacute stroke patients, as there is doubt regarding the ability to detect hyperacute ICH. While a larger number of patients would be useful to confirm these findings, preliminary results suggest that stroke MRI with T2*-WI is as sensitive as CT in the diagnosis of ICH and that there are characteristic features of hyperacute intracerebral hemorrhage on MRI. Also, the combination of PD-WI and FLAIR images may reliably differentiate acute and subacute SAH from ICH and ischemic strokes. In addition, SAH usually presents with a different clinical picture than do ICH and ischemic stroke, unless there is a substantial intracerebral hemorrhage accompanying primary SAH, which then is apparent on T2*-WI. The initial and exclusive use of stroke MRI, therefore, is feasible, cost-effective, and time saving. Thus, stroke MRI may be the diagnostic tool of choice not only for patients with subacute and chronic ICH and SAH but also in the initial assessment of patients with hyperacute ischemic or hemorrhagic stroke as well as hyperacute SAH.

8 Feasibility, Practicality and Logistics of a Multisequence Stroke MRI Protocol

P. D. Schellinger, J. B. Fiebach

The advent of new MRI techniques such as perfusion- (PWI) and diffusion- (DWI) weighted imaging in the early 1990s has added another dimension to diagnostic imaging in stroke [98, 195, 224, 236, 237, 372]. During the last few years a growing body of evidence has accumulated, documenting the usefulness of this method in the clinical setting of acute ischemic stroke. Several investigators found a significant correlation of DWI and PWI changes with follow-up imaging as well as with neurological outcome [18, 205, 322, 344, 371, 373]. Some authors concluded that different infarct patterns can be identified by means of DWI and PWI in hyperacute stroke, which may allow a more rational selection of therapeutic strategies based on the presence or absence of a tissue at risk. Nevertheless, substantial doubts remain regarding the feasibility and practicality as well as the validity of stroke MRI in the clinical setting [268, 397]. In this chapter we discuss the logistic problems that may arise, including solution paths, when this novel methodology is implemented in the clinical routine. Good logistics are the basis for a time efficient diagnosis and treatment process of a stroke patient.

A dedicated stroke service with multimodal imaging availability around the clock (CT, MRI, DSA) requires a sufficiently large staff, infrastructure such as a stroke service, stroke or neurocritical care unit and short distances between emergency room, stroke unit and imaging facilities to save time. At our institution in Heidelberg, for instance, the routine call schedule implies the presence of at least 3 neurology fellows or residents (1 neurointensivist, 1 emergency room neurologist, 1 stroke unit neurologist), 1 neuroradiologist and 1 MR technologist at all times. The MR technologists are familiar with the procedure of stroke MRI, because DWI and PWI are also used in other areas of neuroimaging such as multiple sclerosis and brain tumors [17, 142]. All neuroradiologists have been trained in the use and interpretation of stroke MRI findings. As soon as hyperacute stroke patients are admitted to the emergency room, the neuroradiologist and technician are informed and thus can prepare the infusion pump for PWI as well as the MR scanner while the screening exam, history and stabilization of vital parameters are being performed. Depending on institutional and/or research protocols, CT is also performed (facultatively with CTA and PCT) for, e.g., comparative studies. Ideally, during the day, the patient is directly moved from the CT to the MRI suite or vice versa, which optimally should be next to each other. A CT or MRI examination underway should not be interrupted if only a brief time is needed to finalize the imaging protocol. However, there should be no unnecessary delays in the diagnostic workup as time is of essence in acute stroke patients. At night, when there are no routine MRI procedures being performed, there are no waiting times expected. If there should be a small delay, this can be used to prepare the patient and setup all the monitoring or introduce additional i.v. lines that may be needed. Before being transferred into the MRI suite, the patient and personnel must be checked (check themselves) for any metallic devices in or on his/her body such as surgical scars after pacemaker implantation, coins, piercings, watches, jewelry or others.

At first adequate monitoring has to be performed in the MRI scanner and therefore the treating neurologist or stroke fellow should accompany and care for the patient while the (neuro-) radiologist acquires the scans (Fig. 8.1). Stroke patients should receive 4–8 l O_2 via nasal prongs and the patient's oxygen sat-

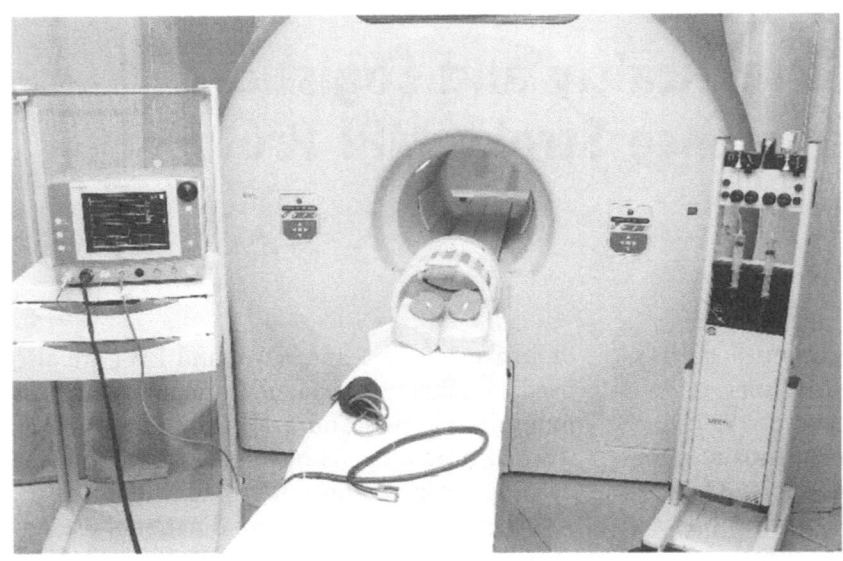

Fig. 8.1. MRI suite with monitor for blood pressure, pulse oxymetry and ECG on the left and infusion pump for PWI on the right. The infusion pump has two syringes, the first for contrast agent and the second for isotonic saline as a flush. In front of the head coil note the foam rubber and ear plugs

uration and ECG should be monitored continuously. If the patient's blood pressure is unstable, the BP can be measured intermittently. All of these monitoring techniques are available as a diagnostic standard in MRI suites. Two aspects with regard to imaging quality of stroke MRI are a major concern, i.e., motion artifacts and noise. Stroke patients can be agitated and restless due to disorientation and aphasia. This, in general, is more pronounced in the more severe stroke patients. Therefore, noise reduction may also help to reduce patient movements. Ear plugs can effectively reduce patient irritation from noise, especially with the EPI sequences. Furthermore, the patient's head can be immobilized with pieces of foam rubber ($5'' \times 2'' \times 8''$), which are stuffed between the head coil and the head on both sides, thus, also adding to the noise reduction achieved by the ear plugs. When the head is immobilized, movement of the non-paretic leg does not influence image quality. Sometimes it may become necessary for the accompanying neurologist to firmly hold the patient's non-paretic hand, because uncooperative patients frequently place it on or into the head coil. When necessary, mild sedation can be given with either propofole 20–60 mg/h continuously i.v. or midazolam 5–10 mg as an i.v. bolus, repeatedly if necessary. In our experience, however, sedation is generally not necessary. A complete stroke MRI protocol

should be comprised of DWI, PWI, MRA, T2-WI and T2*-WI. The net imaging time for a similar protocol is 10 to 15 minutes at maximum and an additional 5 to 10 minutes are necessary for patient positioning and transfer. Calculation of the ADC- and MTT/TTP/CBF-maps should be performed automatically by customized software.

In a pilot study we prospectively recruited acute stroke patients in the 12 h time window for stroke MRI scanning for 2 years (1997–1999) [308]. The basic protocol was designed to identify patients, who are suitable for specific forms of therapy within the first hours of stroke. We included patients with an ischemic stroke within the last 12 hours and a baseline NIHSS score of at least 3, but preferred a time window of 6 hours after symptom onset. Stroke onset in general is defined as the last time the patient was known to be without neurological deficit. All patients had a CT scan before they were enrolled into the MRI study and if thrombolysis was performed this was done with 0.9 mg/kg BW rt-PA in eligible patients with a 6 h time window according to the ECASS II study protocol [126]. To prevent selection bias, the indication for thrombolysis was based exclusively on clinical status and CT findings, not on stroke MRI results. CT was followed by stroke MRI, after which the patient was admitted to the neurocritical care unit, or to the stroke unit for further monitoring and therapy. We examined 64 patients with stroke MRI (mean age 60.9 y, range 29–83 y). The median NIHSS score at baseline was 12 (range 3 to 25) with only 1 patient with a NIHSS score of less than 5. With the exception of 1 patient, the quality of all MRI images obtained was satisfactory for interpretation and without disturbing motion artifacts. One patient did not tolerate the examination despite mild sedation so that only the DWI sequences were interpretable (feasibility = 98.4%). Of the 64 patients included in our study, 25 underwent stroke MRI within 3 hours, 26 within the 3 to 6 h time window and another 13 within the 6 to 12 h time window. The average time of symptom onset to arrival at the neurological emergency room was 2.23 ± 1.64 hours. The mean time from symptom onset to CT was 2.744 ± 1.834 hours, the mean time interval from arrival to CT was 0.603 ± 0.592 hours. The mean time from symptom onset to stroke MRI was 4.48 ± 2.662 hours, from arrival to stroke MRI 2.262 ± 1.949 hours. The mean time interval between CT and stroke MRI was 1.734 ± 1.89 hours. The time window between stroke MRI and CT was significantly reduced with training and growing experience of the involved technical and medical personnel. Before November 1998 as an arbitrarily chosen point of time only 10 of 30 patients received stroke MRI within 1 hour after CT, whereas from November 1998 on 27 of 33 patients underwent stroke MRI within 1 hour after baseline CT ($P = 0.0001$; Chi-square test). Comparing the time intervals before and since November 1998 with the Mann-Whitney U-test, we found a statistically significant difference between the time intervals from symptom onset to stroke MRI ($P = 0.0047$), arrival to stroke MRI ($P = 0.0015$), and between CT and stroke MRI ($P = 0.0007$). The time interval between symptom onset and arrival, as well as that between symptom onset and CT did not differ ($P = 0.48$ and $P = 0.4785$) before and after November 1, 1998. There was a trend but no statistically significant difference in the time interval from arrival to CT ($P = 0.1119$) before and after November 1, 1998. This does not mean, however, that there is no room for improvement with regard to time efficacy. These observations matched our impression that the overall acceptance of

the feasibility and practicality of stroke MRI of those colleagues of the departments of neurology and neuroradiology, who are part of the on-call schedule, had increased decidedly during the study. Subsequently, stroke MRI was successfully implemented as a standard stroke emergency procedure in the clinical routine at all times.

It has been claimed that a method for the selection of patients who benefit most of an effective recanalization therapy would be an improvement [121]. There is a growing body of evidence from many centers that stroke MRI can be performed in an effective and time-saving manner [92, 213, 245, 258–260, 288, 302, 352, 370, 375, 378]. The performance of stroke MRI before initiation of a specific therapy does not lead to an unacceptable loss of time to therapy with a median time window between CT and stroke MRI of one hour. A new diagnostic test must of course show that it can replace a more invasive or more expensive test and that the additional gain in information leads to an improvement of patient management and prognosis [268]. Cost effectiveness of stroke MRI is likely if one considers that multiple examinations such as CT, CTA, and Doppler ultrasound may be substituted by an at least equally accurate imaging modality that is also capable of excluding intracerebral hemorrhage [204, 261, 306]. It is known that optimum stroke care necessitates a lot of manpower [332, 333]. Therefore, in a stroke center there usually are two or more neurologists and an additional neuroradiologist plus a technologist present at all times allowing for the performance of stroke MRI protocols without the need for extra personnel. Furthermore, a gain in information is reached by the substantially higher sensitivity of DWI for stroke location and size [205]. The particular advantage of stroke MRI, however, besides that of rapid demonstration of infarct size and vessel occlusion as the rationale for thrombolytic therapy, is delineation of potential tissue at risk, which represents the aim for most therapeutic efforts [2, 19, 160]. Not only can those patients be identified who profit most from successful recanalization therapy but also those who probably will not, but have an excess risk of complications associated with thrombolysis [328]. However, our and other data show that the time interval to baseline diagnostic imaging (i.e., CT) could not be shortened. Stroke care has to be made a number one public health issue in order to enhance awareness among the population. Time can not only be saved in the clinical workup but also in the preclinical setting [301, 326]. Besides establishing stroke MRI as an initial imaging modality, the time interval from symptom onset or presentation at the emergency room to initial diagnostic imaging must definitely be further reduced. Several multicenter trials to further establish the efficacy and cost benefit ratio of stroke MRI are under way.

In conclusion, stroke MRI is a procedure that rapidly allows a comprehensive diagnostic evaluation of acute stroke patients and provides all necessary and relevant information in the setting of hyperacute stroke. Image quality and information are excellent and can be optimized by head immobilization and by mild sedation, if necessary. Practice and experience with stroke MRI in a stroke team significantly reduces the time effort for this method and facilitates a 24 h availability of stroke MRI. Subsequently, stroke MRI has become part of the clinical routine and thus available 24 h a day on 7 days a week without additional costs for a technologist or physician on call.

9 Comparison of DWI and CT

J.B. Fiebach, P.D. Schellinger

Cerebral ischemia is the leading cause of the acute onset of severe neurological symptoms in stroke patients. Fibrinolysis has become an accepted treatment of cerebral ischemia during the first 3 hours after symptom onset and up to 6 hours in selected cases [125, 304, 305, 338]. The goal of fibrinolytic therapy is to recanalize an occluded basal brain artery and to prevent infarction in a hypoperfused "tissue at risk" [160]. Before initiation of this treatment, however, other causes of acute symptoms such as seizure, encephalitis, and cerebral hemorrhage must be excluded. CT is the imaging modality used most commonly to exclude cerebral hemorrhage. It was also used in the ECASS trial to exclude patients with extensive infarctions from recanalization therapy so as to reduce the incidence of intracranial hemorrhage (ICH) [126]. The main advantage of CT is its widespread availability in many hospitals 24 hours a day. The sensitivity of CT during the first six hours of cerebral ischemia was 64% in the ECASS reading panel with an accuracy of 67%. The local investigators of the ECASS trial only reached a 40% sensitivity (accuracy 45%) [363]. According to the present literature, stroke MRI seems to be the superior imaging modality when compared to CT [16, 18, 302, 344]. All previous studies, however, lack one or more of the following: sufficient patient numbers, blinding of scan interpretation, relevant time window <6 h, preselection of patients not based on the therapeutic target group, and most importantly a negative bias against CT, which was always performed before MRI with a mean time delay averaging 2 hours [92, 113, 191]. Powers and Zivin have addressed the need for a routine means of comparing imaging modalities in ischemic stroke several times [267, 397]. Lansberg and coworkers presented the results of a prospective trial of 19 cerebral infarctions with CT and DWI examination during the first 7 hours of stroke onset. They observed a higher accuracy of DWI for identifying acute infarction and a good sensitivity for detection of infarctions in comparison to CT [191]. The median delay between CT and DWI was 2.5 h, and CT was always performed first. The higher detection rate of DWI was therefore not only based on a different imaging modality but also on the increase in edema over time. In a letter of correspondence, von Kummer criticized the small number of patients in that study and the broad overlap of confidence intervals between the results of CT and DWI [365]. In a pilot study, three neuroradiologists, blinded to clinical signs but aware that they were dealing with stroke, analyzed the CT and DWI of 31 patients with an acute ischemic stroke. The description of interobserver agreement includes unweighted κ-values for blinded interpretation of CT and DWI studies according to Fleiss [99, 190]. In agreement with others, we considered a κ-value below 0.2 as slight, 0.21–0.4 as fair, 0.41–0.6 as moderate, 0.61–0.8 as substantial agreement beyond chance, and 0.81–1 as almost perfect [190, 318, 342, 366]. Sensitivity, specificity, positive and negative predictive values, and accuracy were calculated. The ratings were compared with follow-up studies showing the extent of the infarct. The combined assessment of all observers gave positive findings in 77.4% of all CT examinations, with kappa=0.58. Areas of high signal were seen on all DWI studies by all observers (kappa=1). Estimation of the extent of the infarct based on DWI yielded kappa=0.70 and that based on CT kappa=0.39. DWI was much more reliable than CT in the detection of early ischemic lesions. Also in this pilot study, CT was always performed before stroke MRI, thus, introducing a bias against CT.

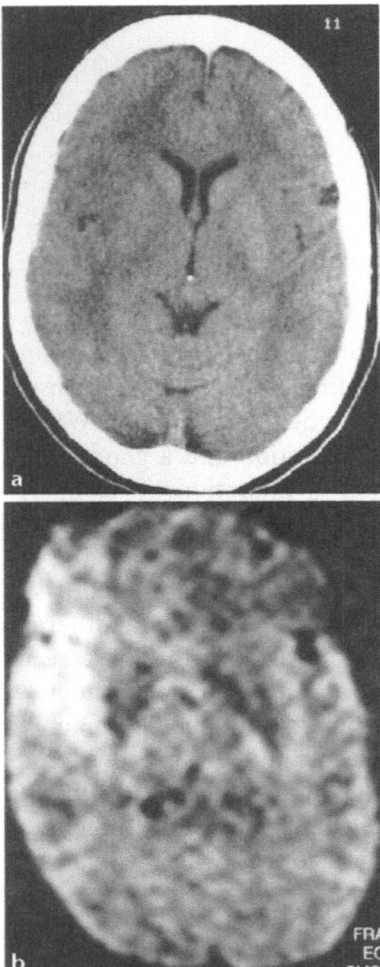

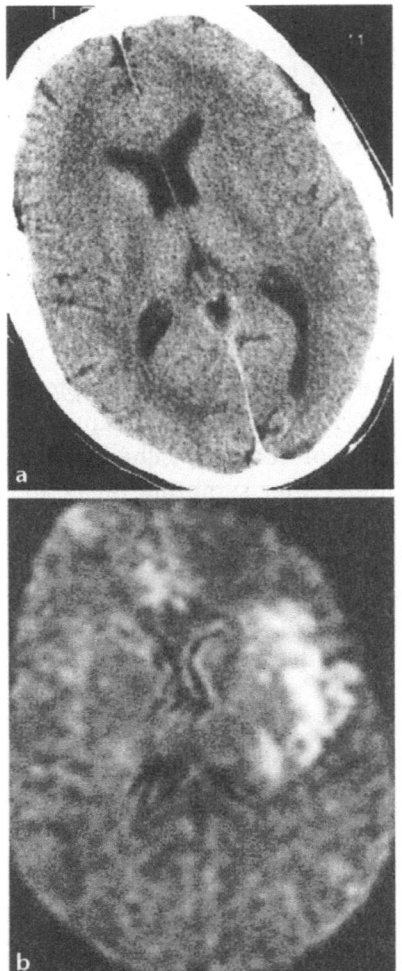

Fig. 9.1. a CT (2 h after symptom onset) and **b** DWI (1 h 43 min after symptom onset) in a patient with a severe hemiparesis and hemihypesthesia on the left side, and hemineglect to the left. There are only minimal early signs of infarction on the CT if any at all. (**a**) The initial rating with clinical background information was sulcal effacement and loss of the gray-white differentiation in the right frontal lobe including the basal ganglia. On DWI (**b**) there is a hyperintensity in the right frontal lobe including part of the frontal insular operculum. MRA showed a M2 occlusion, there was only a small mismatch. The basal ganglia, however, were not included and there was no putaminal infarction on follow-up imaging. CT was less sensitive than DWI and also less specific although it was performed 25 minutes later than DWI

Fig. 9.2. a CT (1 h after symptom onset) and **b** DWI (1 h 15 min after symptom onset) in a patient with a complete left-sided MCA syndrome including hemiplegia on the right side and global aphasia. The CT scan (**a**) is without pathological findings. DWI (**b**) shows a right insular cortex infarction. On MRA there was a proximal M1 occlusion and on PWI there was a corresponding hypoperfusion of the complete MCA territory. The patient received rt-PA 1 h 49 min after symptom onset and did not experience early recanalization, had substantial infarct growth and a poor clinical outcome mRS 4 due to a residual hemiparesis and persistent aphasia

In a new prospective randomized study we compared CT and DWI in hyperacute stroke patients potentially eligible for thrombolytic therapy according to time window and baseline severity of stroke (NIHSS) [94]. To avoid any bias in disfavor of CT due to delay from symptom onset we prospectively randomized our patients to both imaging modalities (either stroke MRI or CT first followed by the other). No images from former studies were included into the analysis so as to avoid any methodological pitfall according to changes in the clinical setting (e. g., dealing with stroke patients in the scanner increasingly becoming a routine procedure). Patients were

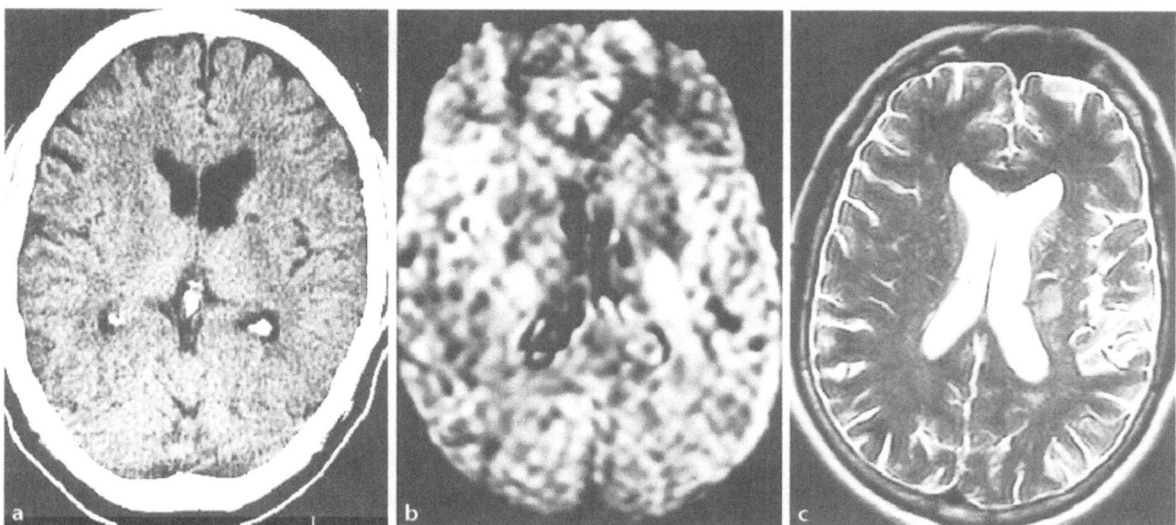

Fig. 9.3. CT (**a**) from a 72-year-old patient 2 h 15 min after onset of a right-sided hemiparesis. There is an old lesion in the left capsule and caudate nucleus but no early sign of a new infarct. DWI (**b**) shows a hyperintensity of the lentiform nucleus in contrast to the CT. The T2-weighted image (**c**) shows the infarction of the lentiform nucleus four days after symptom onset

excluded from further evaluation when the delay from symptom onset to one of the imaging modalities exceeded 6 h or the delay between the two modalities exceeded 90 minutes. After clinical examination, patients were prospectively randomized for the sequence in which the imaging modalities were performed. A total of 20 cases of intracerebral hemorrhage (ICH) and more than 60 ischemic strokes were screened within 6 hours after symptom onset. Patients presented with a median NIHSS score of 11 (range 3–27). In all patients the time of symptom onset could be precisely defined. The correct diagnosis of stroke was established by the clinical course and follow-up CT or MRI examination. Follow-up examinations served as the reference for validation analysis. In total, images from 50 patients with acute brain infarctions and four patients with symptoms of transient ischemic attack (TIA) were included in the analysis. In addition, one case of ICH was introduced as a dummy (Figs. 9.1–9.4).

The scans were read by neurologists and neuroradiologists with considerable experience in stroke imaging. Furthermore, we investigated the accuracy of stroke imaging in a "real-life" clinical setting. Therefore, second and third year residents from the departments of neurology and neuroradiology read the images separately. Early stroke signs on CT, hyperintensities on DWI and lesion extent were judged. Accuracy and sensitivity were calculated for each rater. Finally, we analyzed the interrater variability for both groups in both modalities. The reviewers were unaware of the symptoms and signs the patients had presented with but they knew that the cohort was an ischemic stroke population. All readers were asked to identify and lateralize early stroke signs on CT: presence or absence of loss of the insular ribbon, hypodensity of the lentiform nucleus, focal cortical swelling, and hyperdensity of the middle cerebral artery (MCA) were assessed. The extent of infarction was estimated either in thirds of the MCA territory, as lacunar, or as negative. On DWI, the impaired side and anatomical localization of areas of abnormal, high signal were judged. Again, the readers quantified the extent of the lesion in relation to the MCA territory. The four novices had all read von Kummer's introduction to early stroke signs on CT [364] and were instructed how to deal with the DWI; images from a former study served as examples for typical findings and artifacts [92, 302].

In 54.5% of the study population, DWI was performed first. The mean delay between

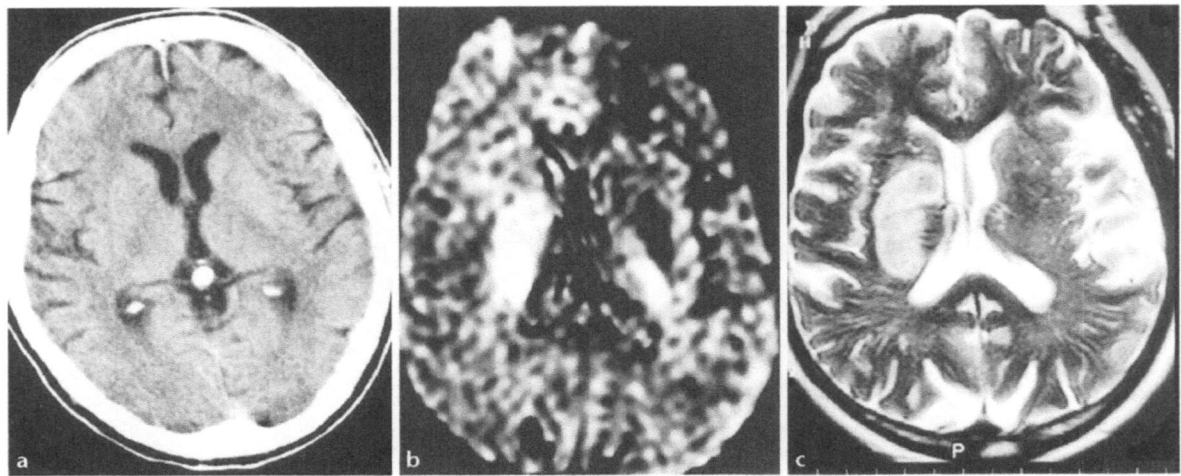

Fig. 9.4. CT (**a**) from a 59-year-old patient 1 h 10 min after onset of a left-sided hemiparesis without pathological findings. DWI (**b**) at 1 h 26 min shows a cortical hyperintensity in contrast to the normal CT findings. Five days after the stroke the T2-weighted image (**c**) shows the subcortical infarction

symptom onset and CT was 180 min, between symptom onset and DWI was 189 min, mean delay between the two examinations was 29 min. All images were of a sufficient diagnostic quality with typical variation according to patient compliance. All the experts identified infarction on 20 CTs reliably. The mean CT sensitivity of the five experts was 61% with a mean specificity of 65%. The accuracy of lesion detection reached 61.8%. Based on early stroke signs the interrater variability for identifying infarctions was $\kappa = 0.51$. Detecting the four early signs of infarction each resulted in a variability of $\kappa = 0.42$–0.52, the estimation of lesion size $\kappa = 0.38$. The median DWI sensitivity of the experts was 91% with a median specificity of 95%. An accuracy of 91.4% was found for lesion detection. The interrater variability was $\kappa = 0.84$ for detecting infarction in general and $\kappa = 0.86$ for hyperintensities of the insular cortex. Rating of hyperintensities of the internal capsule or basal ganglia yielded a value of $\kappa = 0.78$. The positive predictive value was excellent for both modalities (CT/DWI: 96%/100%). For CT, the negative predictive value was 12% (range 9–17%), for DWI 47% (range 38–57%). The homogeneity of stroke detection on DWI increased with the delay from symptom onset.

The novices reached a mean stroke sensitivity of 46% (range 32–64%) on early CT with a specificity of 56%. Accuracy ranged from 35 to 61% (mean 47%). The negative predictive value differed from between 5 and 11% (mean 7%). Mean positive predictive value was 93% (90–96%). Detection of stroke signs showed low homogeneity with $\kappa = 0.38$. Estimation of lesion size was slightly more homogeneous ($\kappa = 0.44$). Readings of the DWI yielded a sensitivity of 78–86% (mean 81%). The homogeneity of lesion detection was high ($\kappa = 0.76$). The novices reached a specificity of 100% (100 %). Mean positive predictive value was 100% (98–100%).

Sensitivity and accuracy of our CT rating (experts) were similar to the results of the experts' rating according to von Kummer in 1996 and as precise as the ECASS II CT reading panel [363, 366]. The assessment of the novices in our study showed a wide variety of sensitivity. The mean sensitivity was slightly higher than that of the ECASS local investigators. The experts' ratings of early stroke signs were as moderately homogeneous as those observed by von Kummer and coworkers [366]. The kappa value of stroke diagnosis based on CT was also moderate. The judgment of lesion size in this study showed fairly good agreement, beyond chance. The sensitivity of DWI was around 91% by the expert raters. No rater reached a 100% detection rate as reported by Lansberg and Gonzáles [113, 191]. Even though DWI changes appear seconds after vessel occlusion in animal models

[286] and cortical hyperintensity was observed in patients 20 min after symptom onset, ischemia might not cause changes on DWI if the hypoperfusion allows structural metabolism. Furthermore, the lesions may also transitorily, partially, or permanently disappear on DWI [173, 243]. The positive predictive value in CT and DWI reached rates of up to 93% in CT and up to 98% in DWI. Compared to Gonzáles et al., we achieved a slightly better result. The false-positive findings on DWI were caused by severe white matter damage. In those cases, the so-called T2-shine through causes a hyperintensity on DWI [270]. Low b-value-DWI, T2-weighted images, or an apparent diffusion coefficient map can be helpful in distinguishing between acute and chronic damage but these options were not offered to the readers [103]. In particular, the selection of clinically thoroughly examined stroke patients with a minimal NIHSS score of 3 prevented a larger number of false-positive findings on DWI. In addition, transient ischemic attacks can cause DWI changes [171]. Recently several groups published results of reversible DWI and ADC changes which did not lead to infarction on follow-up images [95, 171]. As these groups also investigated hyperacute stroke, this discrepancy with our data cannot be explained by different clinical stages of ischemia. However, one difference between the results of those studies and ours with persistent lesions could be how the data were analyzed. We used a standardized presentation of the images with a low window level with a narrow wideness. This means of presenting data could render the extent of a lesion smaller and show sharp margins between healthy tissue and the core of infarction. Therefore, some minor DWI/ADC changes might be missed and only strong hyperintensities considered as infarction. The low negative predictive value of CT judged by the experts can

be taken as proof of the limited prognostic value of CT. The accuracy values of the two modalities prove the superiority of DWI. The interrater variability in infarct detection was excellent for DWI. In a larger cohort such as ours the statistical result is slightly lower than reported for earlier studies. On the other hand, the statistical power with a total number of 55 patients is sufficient. Furthermore, the interrater variability in detecting lesions based on DWI is significantly better.

Comparison between our novices' results and the judgment of the local ECASS II investigators revealed a similar sensitivity. The interrater variabilities of the local ECASS II investigators are not published; however, the novices' ratings show a clinically relevant accuracy. These physicians work nights and weekends. In daily routine, stroke patients should be treated as quickly as possible. In contrast to a study reading panel, no department is able to offer full expert assessment 24 hours a day, 7 days a week as part of clinical routine. Most patients are examined by interns or residents in emergency units during nights and weekends. Under those circumstances the most reliable imaging modality should be used. When a daily stroke MRI routine is established, this modality leads to a short delay between the initial clinical examination and the initiation of therapy [308]. This can also be practiced during nights and weekends.

In conclusion, DWI in hyperacute stroke shows high accuracy and reliability when interpreted even by less experienced physicians. Therefore, DWI should be used instead of CT as the modality of choice in a stroke MRI protocol. Despite the ongoing discussion about reversible changes, DWI shows the infarcted core in nearly every ischemic stroke patient and indicates the actual minimum extension of infarction at the time of imaging in nearly every patient.

10 Characterization of Hyperacute Ischemic Stroke with Stroke MRI

P. D. Schellinger, J. B. Fiebach, S. Warach

In this chapter we will discuss the diagnostic constellations that can be found with stroke MRI in hyperacute stroke patients and how to interpret them. As already stated, within the first few hours, areas of irreversible infarction can be demonstrated reliably on DWI [16, 158, 160, 322, 373] as can ICH [204, 261, 306]. It is presumed that the mismatch between abnormal areas on PWI and DWI (with PWI > DWI) represents the ischemic tissue at risk, which is potentially salvageable from irreversible ischemic damage and may approximate the pathophysiologically defined penumbra [8, 19, 309]. Thus, the term PWI/DWI-mismatch was coined [18, 160, 344]. Conventional sequences such as T2-WI and MRA provide additional information with regard to morphology and vessel status [16, 158]. Several investigators have found a high and significant correlation of changes demonstrated on DWI and PWI with those at follow-up T2-weighted imaging (T2-WI), as well as with neurological outcome as assessed by the NIHSS and the BI [18, 26, 205, 322, 344, 371, 373]. Other authors have proposed that middle cerebral artery (MCA) occlusion predicts a penumbral pattern in combined PWI-DWI [19, 281]. In summary, all these authors concluded that different infarct patterns can be identified by DWI, PWI and MR angiography (MRA) in hyperacute stroke, which may provide us with a more rational selection of therapeutic strategies based on the presence or absence of a tissue at risk for irreversible infarction. Unfortunately, all these studies suffer from one or more of the following: 1) small number of patients; 2) time interval exceeding 6 h after stroke onset; 3) lack of MRA data; and 4) preponderance of mild and less severe strokes.

In a prospective study with a standardized stroke MRI protocol within 6 h after stroke onset and again 24 hours and 5 days thereafter, we examined 51 acute stroke patients at presentation and on days 2, 5, 30 and 90 according to the NIHSS, Scandinavian Stroke Scale (SSS), Modified Rankin Scale (RS), and BI [302]. We introduced DWI, PWI and T2-WI data, PWI/DWI-mismatch, MRA findings, and the clinical presentation and outcome in an analysis to assess and validate the relationship between morphological and clinical deficit as well as the prognostic relevance of stroke MRI. Further, we examined the role of vessel patency or occlusion for further stroke progression, as well as the effects of early recanalization on infarct size and outcome with the ultimate objective of defining patient categories to facilitate treatment decisions. The mean time from symptom onset to arrival at the hospital was 1.86±1.23 hours (range 15 min–4.5 h), from symptom onset to stroke MRI 3.33±1.29 hours (range 1.25–5.75 h), and from CT to MRI 1.035±0.803 hours (range 15 min–3 h 45 min). The time interval in between day 1 and day 2 MRI was 22.41±7.85 hours (range 8.75–34.0 h) and from symptom onset to day 2 MRI 25.73±8.0 hours (range 12.5–38.75 h). We assessed clinical data on days 1, 2, 5, 30 and 90 according to NIHSS [338], SSS [299], BI [211], and RS [272]. We defined a good outcome as a combined endpoint of NIHSS≤1, SSS≥54, BI≥95, MRS≤1 on day 90. In addition, we assessed outcome in a dichotomized fashion with a modified Rankin 0–1 vs 2–6 (favorable vs unfavorable or dead) and modified Rankin 0–2 vs 3–6 (independent vs dependent or dead) in analogy to other studies [126]. We defined a volume ratio of PWI/DWI >1.2 as a relevant perfusion-diffusion mismatch that indicated the presence of tissue at risk. Furthermore, we calculated the difference between PWI and DWI volumes as an absolute measure of tissue at risk. Vessel occlusions were categorized as proximal (distal ICA and proximal M1) or distal (distal M1, M2, A2). Furthermore, we analyzed infarct progression in the following subgroups: patients with persistent occlusion, patients with recanalization after baseline occlusion, and those patients without an occlusion at baseline.

There were 43 patients with a vessel occlusion identified by MRA on day 1: distal ICA occlusion (N = 13), proximal M1 occlusion (N = 12), distal M1 occlusion (N = 8), M2 occlusion (N = 9), and A2 occlusion (N = 1). Eight patients had no occlusion on baseline MRA. Accordingly, 25 patients were included in the proximal occlusion group, 18 patients in the distal occlusion group, and eight patients in the patent group on baseline MRA. Fifteen patients experienced early recanalization (11 of these received thrombolysis, four had a spontaneous vessel reopening). Of the 8 patients without baseline occlusion, 4 had small lacunar infarcts, 2 had basal ganglia infarcts and 2 had presumed small cardioembolic infarcts, 7/8 had no mismatch, 1 patient with a basal ganglia infarct had a very small mismatch ratio of 1.68 (Vol_{DWI} = 8 ml, Vol_{PWI} = 13 ml). The median NIHSS score at presentation was 12±3 (range 3–25), the median SSS score 26±6 (range 4–52). Baseline stroke severity was significantly higher (P = 0.007) in patients with proximal (NIHSS: 9±2; SSS: 23±6) than in those with distal vessel occlusions (NIHSS: 15±4; SSS: 30±5.5). All stroke and outcome scales differed with an increasing level of significance between recanalization and nonrecanalization patients (nonrecanalization patients being worse). In addition, there was a significant difference in the baseline and outcome NIHSS and SSS scores of recanalization patients as opposed to nonrecanalization patients. Furthermore, on day 90 the number of patients with a favorable (MRS 0–1), independent (MRS 0–2), or good (combined endpoint: NIHSS≤1, SSS≥54, BI≥95, MRS≤1) outcome was significantly higher in patients in whom recanalization ensued than in those in whom it did not (all P < 0.0001 except MRS 0–2: P = 0.001; Fisher's exact test). Lesion volumes at baseline (DWI 1) and outcome (T2-WI 5) did not differ in the recanalization group but differed dramati-

cally in the nonrecanalization group with substantial infarct growth between days 2 and 5. There was only a small correlation between baseline lesion volumes and stroke severity which barely reached statistical significance. The correlation only mildly improved in the subgroups, with better correlations of NIHSS and DWI in the recanalization group and of NIHSS and PWI in the nonrecanalization group. Also, DWI 1 and PWI 1 correlated only moderately with NIHSS 90, SSS 90, BI 90, and RS 90 and correlations became worse and nonsignificant for the subgroups. Outcome lesion volumes, however, correlated well and highly significantly with all outcome scores. In 40 patients there was a PWI/DWI-mismatch ratio exceeding 1.2 or 20% on day 1; 39 (97.5%) of these patients had a vessel occlusion according to MRA. Eleven patients had a PWI/DWI-match, seven of whom had a patent vessel. Six patients with a match had lacunar infarcts, another 5 patients had completed ischemic infarction in the vascular territory distal to the occlusion site and then recanalized (N=1) or not (N = 4). The association of vessel occlusion and presence of a mismatch was highly significant (P < 0.0001). On day 2, there were 17 patients with a PWI/DWI-mismatch, 10 of whom also had a vessel occlusion. Of the 20 patients with a patent vessel, only four had a PWI/DWI-mismatch. On day 2 the association of vessel occlusion and presence of a PWI/DWI-mismatch was still significant (P = 0.02). In comparison to day 2 patients with a PWI/DWI-match, the 17 patients with a day 2 mismatch fared worse, as they mostly represented the non-recanalized patients: median day 90 scores RS 3.5 vs. 1; BI 72.5 vs. 90; SSS 35.5 vs. 52; NIHSS 7 vs. 2. The mismatch ratio did not differ between patients with proximal and distal vessel occlusions (P = 0.31); however, the absolute volume at risk did (P = 0.0023). There was a nonsignificant trend towards a higher recanalization rate in patients with distal as opposed to proximal vessel occlusions (P=0.1). Also, clinical outcome was significantly worse in patients with proximal than in those with distal vessel occlusions (combined endpoint: P=0.03; favorable outcome: P=0.001; independent outcome: P=0.002).

It is interesting for the understanding of the relevance of imaging findings whether these findings correlate with the clinical situation. In our study, lesion volumes correlated only moderately with clinical stroke severity at baseline or at outcome. This contradicts the findings of several authors in recent publications, who investigated the correlation of lesion volumes on DWI and PWI with clinical scores at presentation and at outcome, and who consistently reported a high and significant correlation [18, 26, 205, 344, 352]. These five investigators performed stroke MRI in a total of 140 patients, 37 of whom were imaged within 6 h after symptom onset. The most homogeneous study utilizing both, DWI and PWI in 21 hyperacute stroke patients within a mean time to MRI of 5.2 h found high and significant correlations of baseline DWI and PWI volumes with NIHSS at baseline and at 30 days [26]. Although initial stroke severity was fairly similar in the latter study and in ours, our correlation analysis led to strikingly different results. Furthermore, baseline PWI and DWI lesion volumes correlated only modestly with scores at the same timepoint and even worse in the subgroups, which may be partly due to a ceiling effect of the NIHSS, especially in those patients with recanalization, and thus reflects a deficiency of the outcome (i.e., the scale or score) rather than the imaging measure. The less acutely stroke MRI is performed, the more likely it becomes that DWI and PWI findings approximate the final infarct size and thus correlate with clinical outcome which is consistent with older CT and MRI data [45, 226, 298, 361]. Accordingly, day 5 lesion volumes correlated well with clinical outcome. This is also consistent with unpublished data from other groups (P. A. Barber, Royal Melbourne Hospital, Australia, personal communication). Therefore, we assume that our findings are consistent with those of others, who performed imaging at a later time when infarct dynamics are not an issue anymore. In the hyperacute stage of stroke, however, the baseline DWI and PWI lesion size neither reflect the clinical degree of severity at baseline nor at outcome, but rather illustrate the potential best and worse case scenarios. The clinical and morphological course of hyperacute ischemic infarction is completely open and thus may be influenced by therapy. Therefore the mismatch and the evaluation of best or worse outcome should be used to differentiate which patients are at a high risk and which are not. Stroke MRI findings are far more reliable in predicting what fate the patient *may* face if not treated (final stroke size ≈ PWI size) or effectively treated (final stroke size ≈ DWI size).

Also it is important to understand to what extent the vascular status corresponds to patient prognosis and imaging findings. Furthermore, assessment of the vascular status allows validation of the findings on DWI and PWI. Rordorf et al. investigated 17 patients with combined MRA, DWI and PWI within 12 h after symptom onset [281]. Of the patients with an occluded MCA, 70% had a PWI/DWI-mismatch, and all of them had infarcts at outcome that were larger than the baseline DWI lesion as compared to the seven patients without vessel occlusion. Barber et al. published the findings from 26 patients in whom stroke MRI was performed within 24 h after symptom onset and reported a significant association of vessel occlusion and a PWI/DWI-mismatch [19]. While we agree with the conclusions of both groups, we believe that due to the rather late imaging time in some of their patients either spontaneous or therapeutic recanalization had already occurred. We found a baseline vessel occlusion in 84% of our patients as opposed to 35% [19] and 58% [281], respectively. The association of vessel occlusion and PWI/DWI-mismatch (97.5%) and vessel patency and PWI/DWI-match (64%) was strikingly significant, especially when considering that the remaining four patients with vessel occlusion and PWI/DWI-match had completed their infarction without experiencing recanalization. As others, we observed only a statistical trend towards a smaller recanalization rate with more proximal vessel occlusions, which with larger patient numbers eventually may reach statistical significance (Figs. 10.1–10.3) [161, 367, 395].

An interesting observation also shared by others is the persistence of a PWI/DWI-mismatch even more than 24 hours after stroke onset [19, 281]. This may imply that even recanalization after one day may be beneficial for a patient with tissue at risk and a persisting vessel occlusion. Recanalization later than

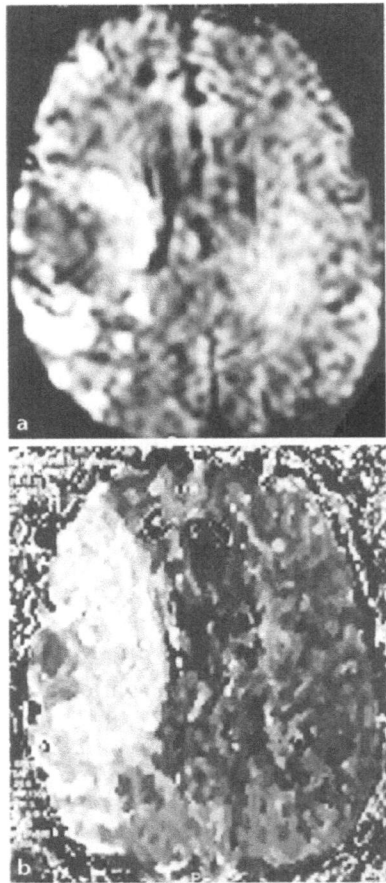

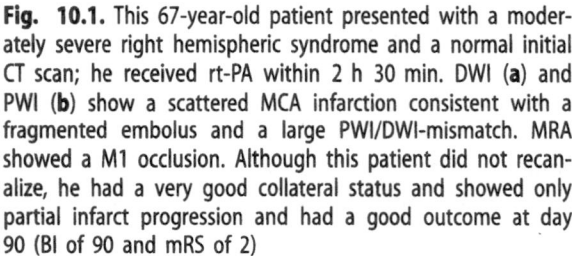

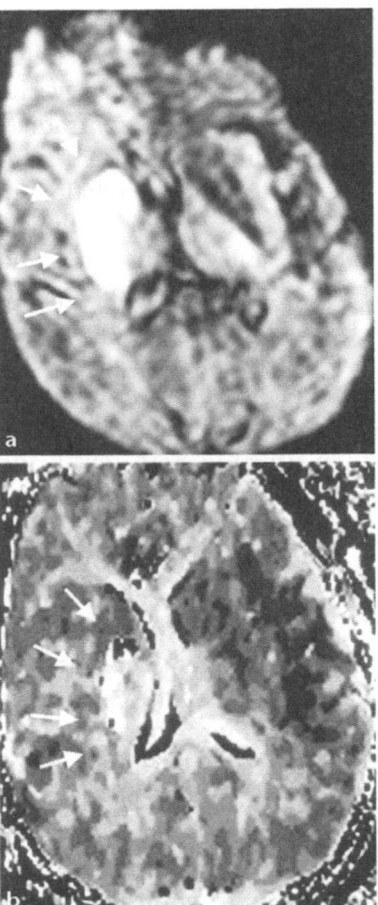

Fig. 10.1. This 67-year-old patient presented with a moderately severe right hemispheric syndrome and a normal initial CT scan; he received rt-PA within 2 h 30 min. DWI (**a**) and PWI (**b**) show a scattered MCA infarction consistent with a fragmented embolus and a large PWI/DWI-mismatch. MRA showed a M1 occlusion. Although this patient did not recanalize, he had a very good collateral status and showed only partial infarct progression and had a good outcome at day 90 (BI of 90 and mRS of 2)

Fig. 10.2. A 59-year-old man with arterial hypertension and obesity presenting 1 h 26 min after symptom onset. He had a moderately severe left-sided hemiparesis. DWI (**a**) shows an ischemic infarction of the basal ganglia as a hyperintense lesion. PWI (**b**) also shows a hyperintensity corresponding in size to the lesion on DWI (*arrows*). This patient has a perfusion-diffusion match

8 hours after stroke onset has been shown to improve patient outcome [367]. Also, a protracted metabolic recovery after thrombolysis may still be associated with a good clinical result [32]. On the other hand, intravenous thrombolysis later than 3 h and intraarterial thrombolysis later than 6 h, while clinically highly effective when recanalization is achieved, have failed to prove efficacious [66, 70, 102, 125, 126, 338]. In our patients, a day 2 mismatch was present only in the patients without recanalization and therefore associated with a poor outcome. We believe that recanalization at such a late point of time will

have a small effect at best and has to be weighed against the risk of reperfusion injury including fatal ICH. Another study found a high number of patients with a relevant mismatch (93%) and with vessel occlusion in MRA (90%) in their cohort of 139 patients [288]. Patients without mismatch were likely to present with spontaneous recanalization, lacunar infarcts, or large, scarcely collateralized hemispheric infarcts due to proximal vessel occlusions. These authors also found two subgroups in their population of 19 patients without a relevant mismatch that support this view: the first subgroup (n = 8) had

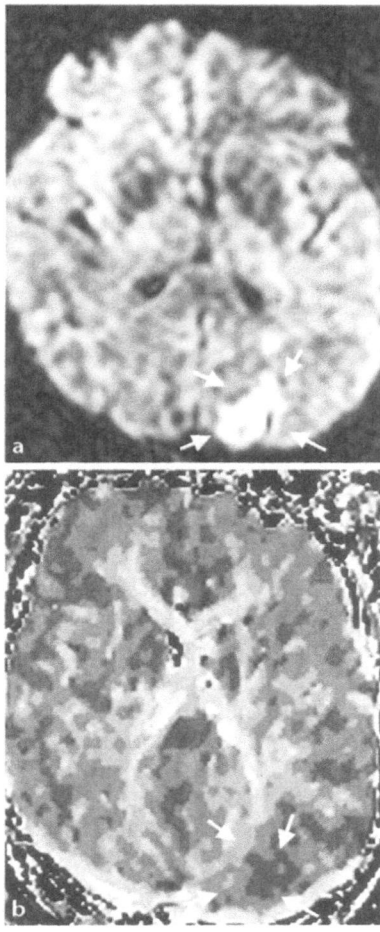

Fig. 10.3. This patient suffered a hemisensory stroke with hemianopia and minimal aphasia. DWI (**a**) shows the left occipital infarction as a hyperintensity; PWI (**b**) is normal if not hyperperfused. This patient experienced complete recanalization with non-nutritional reperfusion

small initial DWI lesion and final infarct volumes, patent vessels and normal PWI. These patients, who had either lacunar strokes or spontaneously recanalized peripheral branch occlusions, had good functional outcomes. The other subgroup presented with large DWI and PWI lesion volumes and MCA or carotid artery occlusions. Even at a very early imaging time (210 minutes after stroke onset), patients had no relevant mismatch and accordingly developed large final infarct volumes and poor functional outcomes. More data are needed before recommendations for aggressive therapeutic procedures such as late i.v. or i.a. thrombolysis or early hemicraniectomy or hypothermia based on a persisting PWI/

DWI-mismatch can be given [313–315]. Preliminary data on the power of stroke MRI to predict malignant MCA infarction have been published by Oppenheim et al. [255]. Out of 28 patients with a MCA infarct and proven MCA or carotid T occlusion on DWI and MRI angiography performed within 14 hours after onset (mean 6.5±3.5 hours, median 5.2 hours), 10 patients developed malignant MCA infarct, whereas 18 did not. Univariate analysis showed that an admission NIHSS score >20, total versus partial MCA infarct, and volume (DWI) >145 ml were highly significant predictors of malignant infarct. The best predictor was DWI volume, which achieved 100% sensitivity and 94% specificity. Prediction was further improved by bivariate models combining DWI volume and ADC measurements, which reached 100% sensitivity and specificity in this series of patients. Further data are pending.

Although evidence of DWI lesion reversibility is accumulating, we did not observe this in any of our patients. However, other reports differ from ours in that they either presented experimental data [203], individual observations [235], patients with transient ischemic attacks [171], or patients, who received intraarterial thrombolytic therapy with rt-PA or urokinase and experienced "ultraearly" recanalization [173] (Fig. 10.4). In 3/7 patients in the latter study, however, the lesions reappeared [173]. While these findings and those of other groups [57, 300] qualify the rather rigid dogma of only the PWI/DWI-mismatch representing tissue at risk for irreversible infarction and non-reversibility of DWI lesions, we believe that only a minority of patients with either very mild strokes, transient ischemic attacks, or "ultraearly" recanalization will have reversible ischemic damage in an area seen as a lesion on DWI. On the other hand, if only a small area of DWI disturbance is not turning into an irreversible lesion, this may improve the clinical outcome of an individual patient and therefore has to be taken into account when making treatment decisions.

Another important issue is the effect of early recanalization on PWI and DWI lesions and clinical outcome. In one study, five out of six patients, who had received rt-PA and un-

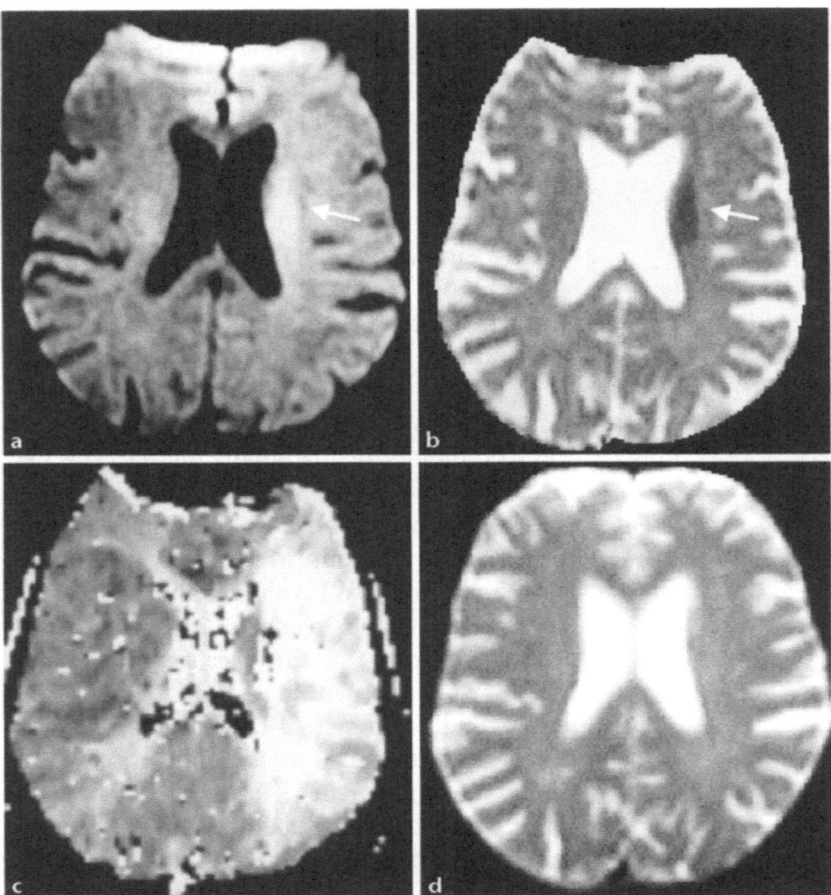

Fig. 10.4. This 60-year-old patient had a non-fluent aphasia and hemiparesis on the right side. MRA showed a M1 occlusion, the patient received rt-PA within 2 hours after symptom onset and experienced early recanalization. DWI (**a**, *arrow*) shows a hyperintensity adjacent to the left lateral ventricle also seen as a hypointensity or ADC decrease in the ADC map (**b**, *arrow*). PWI shows a hypoperfusion of the complete left MCA territory consistent with M1 occlusion (**c**). At day 7, the T2-WI (**d**) is without pathological findings. This is a rare example of reversal of a DWI/ADC lesion (courtesy of J. Fiehler, MD, Dept. of Neurology, University Clinic at Hamburg, Germany)

derwent stroke MRI thereafter, had smaller PWI than DWI volumes, suggesting early recanalization [213]. Jansen et al. published a series of 35 patients and concluded that early recanalization may save tissue at risk of infarction as defined by DWI and PWI [160]. This is consistent with findings from early angiography and more recent DU studies [5, 62, 277, 278]. Another series with a substantially larger number of patients imaged at an earlier timepoint offers strong evidence in support of the latter study: early recanalization in patients with a baseline vessel occlusion is associated with a dramatically better outcome at days 30 and 90 in four clinical scales alone and in combination with a dichotomized analysis. The morphological course of ischemic infarction parallels the clinical course. With regard to the controversly discussed utility of stroke MRI [267], we believe that the constellation of the DWI,

PWI, MRA, T2-WI and PWI/DWI-mismatch allows the early identification of those patients in whom outcome and final infarct size, ultimately the patient's fate, have not yet been determined. Furthermore, stroke MRI may be useful in identifying those patients not suitable for thrombolysis because of extensive infarctions [128], and those with large infarctions and a PWI/DWI-mismatch, which might be salvaged by more aggressive means [276, 314, 315].

In summary, hyperacute DWI and PWI lesion volumes correlate only modestly with clinical stroke severity at the same point in time or at outcome since the infarct dynamics in hyperacute stroke <6 h, reflecting the clinical observation that the patient's fate has not been decided yet. Early recanalization saves tissue at risk of ischemic infarction, as shown by resolution of a PWI/DWI-mismatch, and results in significantly smaller infarcts and a significantly better clinical outcome. In patients with proximal vessel occlusions, a larger area of tissue is at risk, the recanalization rate is lower, and outcome is worse, and, therefore, vessel patency should be achieved by all means in this patient group. Vessel occlusion predicts presence of a PWI/DWI-mismatch. While in most instances DWI lesions represent irreversibly damaged brain tissue, these lesions may be in part reversible when stroke is treated early and effectively.

11 Thrombolytic Therapy in Stroke

P. D. Schellinger, W. Hacke

Up to 85% of all strokes are of ischemic origin and mostly due to blockage of a cerebral artery by a blood clot [129, 388]. After introduction of thrombolytic therapy for the treatment of acute myocardial infarction in the early 1990s [335], major trials for the evaluation of this new therapeutic approach to ischemic stroke were initiated. Occlusion of a brain vessel leads to a critical reduction in cerebral perfusion and, within minutes, to ischemic infarction with a central infarct core of irreversibly damaged brain tissue and an area of variable size of hypoperfused but still vital brain tissue (the ischemic penumbra), which can potentially be salvaged by rapid restoration of blood flow [8, 130]. Therefore, the underlying rationale for the introduction and application of thrombolytic agents is the lysis of a thrombus and subsequent reestablishment of cerebral blood flow by cerebrovascular recanalization [132]. The local delivery of thrombolytic agents, at or within the thromboembolism, has the advantage of providing a higher concentration of the particular thrombolytic agent where it is needed while minimizing the concentration systemically. Hence, local intra-arterial thrombolysis has the potential for greater efficacy with higher arterial recanalization rates and greater safety with lower risk of hemorrhage. The technique involves performing a cerebral arteriogram, localizing the occluding clot, navigating a microcatheter to the site of the clot, and administering the lytic agent at or inside the clot with or without mechanical destruction of the thrombus. Grade of vessel occlusion is usually assessed with the Thrombolysis in Myocardial Infarction (TIMI) score, where TIMI 0 is complete occlusion, TIMI 1 minimal perfusion, TIMI 2 partial flow (recanalization), and TIMI 3 complete flow (recanalization) [339]. The agents most commonly used or which are under investigation are urokinase, t-PA (alteplase), and pro-urokinase, all of which are usually administered at a lower dose than used in the intravenous treatment of acute ischemic stroke.

◾ Randomized Trials of Intravenous Thrombolysis

The first anecdotal report of thrombolytic therapy for ischemic stroke dates back to the early 1960s [222]. Three trials in the early 1980s investigated the effect of low-dose intravenous urokinase for the therapy of acute ischemic stroke [1, 9, 253]. These trials differ from others for several reasons, such as a late timepoint of inclusion (up to 5 or 14 days after stroke onset, respectively), the exclusion of presumed cardioembolic stroke, application of low doses of urokinase given daily for a period of several days, and the lack of assessment of clinical outcome except death and ICH. In the early 1990s three small trials of intravenous thrombolysis with rt-PA were carried out, two of them in Japan [137, 232, 391]. Although not large enough to prove the efficacy, they clearly showed the feasibility of early thrombolytic therapy and also suggested a reasonable degree of safety and a potential benefit. All these trials were blinded or double-blinded, randomized, and placebo-controlled.

One pilot study and three large trials investigated the efficacy of streptokinase for acute ischemic stroke [83, 234, 336, 337]. In summary, all of the trials using streptokinase for acute ischemic stroke were prematurely stopped due to a high rate of early death, mostly due to ICH, and because of a lack of benefit at outcome in a meta-analysis [72]. In the streptokinase trials together there were 92 (95% CI 65 to 120) additional fatal ICH per 1000 treated patients (OR 6.03, 95% CI 3.47 to 10.47) [379]. The higher bleeding rate may be due to pharmacological properties of streptokinase other than, for instance, rt-PA, additional anticoagulation (MAST-E), a rather small fraction of patients treated within 3 hours, and a rather high dose of 1.5 MU, which is identical to the dose used in myocardial infarction (MI), whereas the rt-PA studies (see below) chose approximately two thirds the dose used in MI. Other side effects of streptokinase are a decrease in systolic blood pressure of more than 20 mmHg in 33% (only 6% in the placebo group) as well as anaphylaxis in 2.2% of the patients. Therefore, intravenous administration of streptokinase, outside the setting of a clinical investigation, is dangerous and not indicated for the management of patients with ischemic stroke.

In 1995, the results of the ECASS I and NINDS trials of intravenous rt-PA for acute ischemic stroke were published [125, 338] and followed by ECASS II in 1998 [126] and ATLANTIS in 1999 [70]. These 4 trials randomized a total of 2657 patients to treatment with placebo (N = 1316 patients) or intravenous rt-PA (N = 1341 patients) within 0–3 hours (NINDS), 3–5 hours (ATLANTIS), or 0–6 hours (ECASS I and II) after symptom onset. All four studies required a baseline CT scan to exclude ICH, and except for the NINDS study all others also established CT exclusion criteria such as major early signs of infarction. All trials used the 0.9 mg/kg bodyweight dose up to a maximum of 90 mg rt-PA, except ECASS I, in which 1.1 mg/kg up to a maximum dose of 100 mg was given. Ten percent of the total dose was given as a bolus; the rest was infused over 1 hour in all 4 trials.

The NINDS trial randomized 624 patients (312 each placebo and intravenous rt-PA) within a time window of 3 hours after stroke symptom onset [338]. Half of the patients were treated within 0–90 minutes, the other half within 91–180 minutes. A good outcome was defined as a NIHSS score of ≤1, GOS = 1, BI ≥95, and MRS ≤1. The median baseline NIHSS score was 14 (rt–PA group) versus 15 (placebo group). There was no significant difference between the drug treatment and pla-

cebo group in the percentages of patients with neurologic improvement at 24 hours (rt-PA 47% versus placebo 57%; RR 1.2, P = 0.21), although a post hoc analysis comparing the median NIHSS scores at 24 hours showed a median of 8 in the rt-PA-treated group versus 12 in the placebo group (P <0.02). Furthermore, a benefit was observed for the t-PA group at 3 months for all four outcome measures. The long-term clinical benefit of t-PA was confirmed in all single scores as well as in the global test: BI (50% vs 38%, OR 1.6 (1.1–2.5), P = 0.026); MRS (39% vs 26%, OR 1.7 (1.1–2.5), P = 0.019); GOS (44% vs 32%, OR 1.6 (1.1–2.5), P = 0.025); NIHSS (31% vs 20%, OR 1.7 (1.0–2.8), P = 0.033); and combined endpoint (OR 1.7 (1.2–2.6), P = 0.008). For every 100 patients treated with rt-PA, an additional 11 to 13 will have a favorable outcome as compared to 100 not treated with rt-PA. Outcome did not vary by stroke subtype at baseline, meaning that patients with small vessel disease benefited as well as patients with, for instance, cardioembolic stroke. On the other hand, small vessel disease was clinically defined and not identified by imaging studies. Symptomatic ICH within 36 hours after the onset of stroke occurred in 6.4% of patients given t-PA but only in 0.6% of patients given placebo (P <0.001). Nevertheless, severe disability and death were higher in the nontreated group (mortality at 3 months: t-PA 17% versus placebo 21%, P = 0.30). After publication of the NINDS trial in 1996, rt-PA received FDA approval for the treatment of acute ischemic stroke in a time window of 3 hours.

ECASS I, a prospective, multicenter, randomized, double-blind, placebo-controlled trial, recruited 620 patients for treatment either with 1.1 mg/kg rt-PA or placebo within 6 hours after stroke symptom onset [125]. Anticoagulants, neuroprotectants, and rheologic therapy were prohibited during the first 24 hours. Patients with a severe deficit (hemiplegia, forced head and eye movement, and impairment of consciousness), with only mild or improving stroke symptoms, or CT signs of early infarction exceeding 33% of the middle cerebral artery (MCA) territory were excluded. Primary endpoints included a difference of 15 points in the BI and 1 point in the MRS at 90 days in favor of rt-PA. Secondary endpoints included combined BI and MRS, Scandinavian Stroke Scale (SSS) at 90 days, and 30-day mortality. In anticipation of a substantial number of protocol violations due to the first time that early CT signs of infarction were being used as an inclusion criterion, the investigators prospectively specified a target population (TP) analysis in addition to the primary intention to treat (ITT) analysis, which was performed at the end of the trial. The median NIHSS score at baseline was 13 (rt-PA patients) and 12 (placebo group), respectively. ECASS I was the first trial of thrombolysis to use CT exclusion criteria [360, 361, 368, 369]. In spite of these predefined parameters, there were 109 protocol violations in ECASS I (17.4%), 66 (11%) of which were CT protocol violations and 52 (8.4%) of these due to maldetection of early infarct signs. There was no difference in the primary endpoints in the ITT analysis, while the TP analysis revealed a significant difference in the MRS (but not BI) in favor of rt-PA-treated patients (P = 0.035). Of the secondary endpoints, the combined BI and RS showed a difference in favor of rt-PA-treated patients (P < 0.001). Neurologic recovery at 90 days was significantly better for rt-PA-treated patients in the TP (P = 0.03). There was a nonsignificant trend towards a higher mortality rate at 30 days (P = 0.08) and a significant increase in parenchymal ICH (19.8% versus 6.5%, P < 0.001). There was a significant inverse relationship between protocol violation in rt-PA patients and 7-day survival. A post hoc analysis of the ECASS I 3-hour cohort (N = 87 patients) did not reveal a significant difference between rt-PA and placebo group outcomes [325].

ECASS II randomized a total of 800 patients (409 rt-PA, 391 placebo) to treatment with either 0.9 mg/kg rt-PA or placebo within 6 hours (stratified into a 0–3 hour and a 3–6 hour group) after stroke symptom onset [126]. The primary endpoint was the MRS at 90 days, dichotomized for favorable (score 0–1) and unfavorable (score 2–6) outcome. Analyses were by ITT and an 8% absolute difference was aimed for in the primary endpoint. Secondary endpoints were a combined BI and MRS at day 90 and the NIHSS at day 30. A post hoc analysis requested by the board of reviewers was performed for an alternative dichotomization into independent versus death and dependent outcome (MRS 0–2 versus 3–6). Baseline median NIHSS was 11 in both groups, which is 2–3 points less than in NINDS and ECASS I. The safety analysis showed a similar mortality in the two groups (10.5% versus 10.7%): there was a substantially larger number of fatal ICH in the rt-PA group (11 versus 2 patients), whereas more patients died due to space-occupying brain edema (8 versus 17 patients). There was a fourfold increase in symptomatic parenchymal ICH (48 versus 12 patients) in the rt-PA group, which was a far lower rate than in ECASS I. The primary endpoint was negative for rt-PA (MRS 0.1: 40.3% versus 36.6%; Δ = 3.7%; P = 0.277). There was a trend for the combined BI/MRS endpoint (P = 0.098) and a significant difference in the day 30 NIHSS score (P = 0.035). With the alternative dichotomization, a significant advantage for patients treated with rt-PA (MRS 0–2: 54.3% vs. 46.0%; Δ = 8.3%; P = 0.024) was demonstrated. Like in ECASS I, the 3 h cohort did not show any significant differences due to the small patient numbers (N = 80 patients/group). Symptomatic ICH occurred in 36 (8.8%) rt-PA patients and 13 (3.4%) placebo-treated patients. Interestingly, there was a high number of benign spontaneous disease courses in the placebo group (36.6%), which is larger than the favorable outcome rate in the ECASS I rt-PA group (35.9%). Furthermore, a comparison of the 3 h cohorts of ECASS I and II and NINDS demonstrates a surprisingly high number of favorable outcomes among the placebo group patients in ECASS II (ECASS I rt-PA: 38.5%; NINDS rt-PA: 38.7%; ECASS II placebo: 37.7%). Whether this is due to general improvements in the treatment of acute stroke patients, a less severe baseline deficit, or other factors is unclear. While negative for the primary endpoint, ECASS II was a clinically highly relevant study and showed that treatment of ischemic stroke with rt-PA in a time window of less than 6 hours may lead to an improved outcome if given to selected patients in experienced centers.

The ATLANTIS study began in 1991 and was originally designed to assess efficacy and safety of thrombolytic therapy with rt-PA within 0–6 hours after stroke symptom onset [70]. In 1993, the time window was changed due to safety concerns to 0–5 hours and re-started as part B (ITT), only to be further modified in 1996 to a 3–5 hour window (TP) after rt-PA had been approved by the FDA. Part A enrolled 142 patients (22 <3 hours; 46 >5 hours) [66]. The primary endpoint was an improvement of 4 or more points on the NIHSS at 24 hours and day 30; secondary endpoints included functional outcome (BI and MRS) at days 30 and 90. There was a significant improvement at 24 hours in the rt-PA group (40% versus 21%, P=0.02); this effect, however, was reversed at day 30 (60% versus 75%, P=0.05). rt-PA significantly raised the rate of symptomatic ICH (11% versus 0%, P <0.01) and mortality at 90 days (23% versus 7%, P <0.01). The primary endpoint for part B was a NIHSS score of ≤1 at 90 days; secondary endpoints were outcome at days 30 and 90 according to BI, MRS, and GOS. An ITT population of 613 acute ischemic stroke patients was enrolled, with 547 of these treated as assigned within 3 to 5 hours of symptom onset (TP). There were no differences on any of the primary (34% versus 32%, P=0.65) or secondary functional outcome measures; however, there was a significant difference in the rate of major neurologic recovery (complete or ≥11 NIHSS points improvement: 44.9% versus 36%, P=0.03), which did not affect overall outcome. Treatment with rt-PA significantly increased the rate of symptomatic ICH (7.0% versus 1.1% P <0.001). As in ECASS II (median baseline NIHSS: 11 points), the median baseline NIHSS score was substantially lower than in the NINDS trial (10 versus 14 points), which (as in ECASS II) may have led to a better than expected outcome in the placebo group. In contrast to ECASS II, ATLANTIS was negative for the alternate outcome measurement independence (MRS 0–2) versus dependence or death (MRS 3–6) (rt-PA 54% versus placebo 56%, P=0.75). The authors conclude that thrombolysis with r-PA for acute ischemic stroke later than 3 hours after symptom onset cannot be recommended.

Meta-analyses

A search of the literature revealed two large meta-analyses [124, 379, 380]. The first meta-analysis by Hacke et al. from 1999 [124] covered the NINDS study and both ECASS trials, with a total of 2044 patients included (1034 rt-PA patients versus 1010 placebo patients). The authors assessed the benefit of rt-PA by dichotomizing the outcome into dependent versus independent or dead (MRS 0–2 versus 3–6) and favorable versus unfavorable (MRS 0–1 versus MRS 2–6). Risk in these three trials can be defined as ICH and mortality. Differences between the trials such as the dose of rt-PA (1.1 mg/kg in ECASS I versus 0.9 mg/kg in NINDS and ECASS II) and the therapeutic time window (3 hours in NINDS versus 6 hours in ECASS I and II) were taken into account. ICH occurred significantly more often in patients receiving rt-PA (144/1034 versus 43/1010; OR 3.23, CI 2.39–4.37), and was slightly less increased in the 3 h time window and at the lower dosage (41/393 versus 15/389; OR 2.68, CI 1.56–4.62). There was no significant difference in mortality between rt-PA and placebo (OR 1.07, CI 0.84–1.36) but a slight trend towards a lower mortality in the 0.9 mg/kg and 3 h group (OR 0.91, 0.63–1.32). rt-PA, on the other hand, led to a 37% reduction in death and dependence regardless of dose and time window (OR 0.63, CI 0.53–0.76). If treated with the lower dose and within 3 hours, the chance of an unfavorable outcome was reduced by 45% (OR 0.55, CI 0.41–0.72). For every 1000 patients treated with either dose, there are 90 fewer patients who are dead or disabled but 96 hemorrhages more than expected with placebo. Conversely, for 1000 patients treated with 0.9 mg/kg and within 3 hours, there are 65 additional ICH and 140 fewer patients dead or disabled. The NNT for all doses and time windows is 11; for the 3 h and 0.9 mg/kg group it is 7. These numbers are far better than the NNT for thrombolysis in myocardial infarctions, which is 30–40 [124].

Wardlaw et al. included in their Cochrane Library meta-analysis all randomized trials of thrombolysis regardless of time window, dosage, administration route, and substance [379, 380]. Seventeen trials with a total of 5216 patients (2889 of which were from rt-PA trials) were included. The 17 trials were NINDS, ECASS I and II, ATLANTIS A and B (with preliminary data), PROACT I and II (with preliminary data), ASK, MAST-E, MAST-I, and the early trials by Abe, Atarashi, Haley, Mori, Morris, Ohtomo, and Yamaguchi [1, 9, 66, 70, 80, 83, 102, 125, 126, 137, 232, 234, 253, 336–338, 391]. The main objectives were to show that thrombolytic therapy reduces the risk of late death, increases the risk of early and fatal ICH, and that the benefit at outcome (reduction of death and dependence) offsets any early hazard. Symptomatic and fatal ICH were significantly more common as a result of thrombolytic therapy (symptomatic ICH: OR 3.53, CI 2.79–4.45, P < 0.000001; fatal ICH: OR 4.15, CI 2.96–5.84). This translates into 70 additional instances of symptomatic ICH for patients receiving thrombolysis and 29/1000 (OR 3.2) additional instances of fatal ICH in rt-PA patients but 92/1000 (OR 6.03) additional ICH in those patients receiving streptokinase as opposed to placebo. Despite this, thrombolytic therapy, administered up to 6 hours after ischemic stroke, significantly reduced death or dependence at the end of follow-up (55.2% versus 59.7%, OR 0.83, CI 0.73 to 0.94, P = 0.0015), which is equivalent to 44 fewer patients being dead or dependent per 1000 treated (CI 15–73). For patients treated with rt-PA only, the OR was 0.79 (CI 0.68–0.92, P = 0.001) or 57 deaths/dependence prevented per 1000 patients treated (CI 20–93). An alternative endpoint analysis yields similar results for favorable versus unfavorable outcome (OR 0.79 for all patients and 0.76 for rt-PA patients). When treatment was given within 3 hours after stroke onset, there was an even better risk reduction for dependency or death (55.2% versus 68.3%; OR 0.58, CI 0.46 to 0.74, P = 0.00001) or 126 fewer dead or dependent patients per 1000 treated. The difference of benefit of rt-PA in the 0–3 hour window or 3–6 hour window was nonsignificant but showed a trend towards better improvement with early therapy (OR 0.7 versus 0.76). The authors conclude that the significant increase in early death and fatal and nonfatal symptomatic ICH are offset by the significant reduction of disability in survivors. Therapy with

rt-PA is associated with less risk and more benefit than with other substances.

Recently, Brott presented a new meta-analysis of the NINDS, ECASS I and II and ATLANTIS studies in San Antonio at the American Stroke Association meeting [46]. They quadrotomized the time interval to treatment in 90 minutes intervals (0–90; 91–180; 181–270; 271–360 min) and analyzed the ratio of patients with a favorable outcome (mRS 0–1) in 2776 patients (Fig. 11.1). They found a significant correlation of outcome with time from symptom onset. The odds ratios for the favorable outcome were 2.83, 1.53, 1.4 and 1.16 respectively with the last OR missing statistical significance. The lower confidence interval intersects with 1.0 at 285 minutes after symptom onset. Interestingly, the significant effect in favor of rt-PA is mainly on the cost of patients in the mRS range from 2–5 but there is no difference in death (mRS 6). Thus, the negative correlation of time loss with outcome is again established ("Time is Brain").

A stroke MRI-based study on the efficacy of recombinant desmoteplase (DSPA, derived from saliva of the vampire bat *Desmodus rotundus*) for treatment of stroke in the 3–9 hour time window has resumed recruitment after having been on halt due to safety concerns (DIAS = Desmoplase In Acute ischemic Stroke). A pilot trial with tenecteplase (TNK) for acute ischemic stroke is planned. DEFUSE (USA) and EPITETH (Australia) are two studies that perform MRI-based thrombolysis with rt-PA in the 3–6 h time window, data are currently not available. IST 3 is a large thrombolysis trial planned to include thousands of patients in a randomized fashion with the uncertainty principle. This means that physicians who want to treat their patients with rt-PA should do so, those that do not want to treat a specific patient should not. However, when not being sure whether to treat or not they should randomize the patient. We believe that the Cleveland area experience has clearly demonstrated that physicians, who do not know whom to treat and whom not to treat should not use rt-PA as there will be an abundance of hemorrhagic complications [170]. However, another trial of rt-PA for ischemic stroke – ECASS III – has

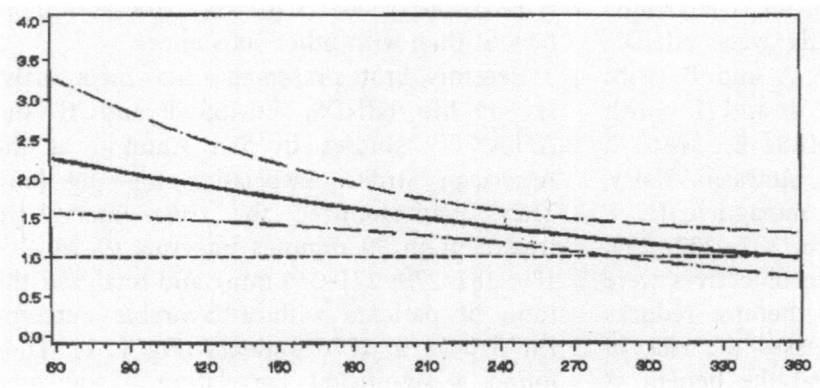

Fig. 11.1. Treatment effect of thrombolysis over time

been demanded by the European authorities and is currently in the planning phase. As many patients do not arrive in the hospital within 3 hours, the aim of ECASS III is to extend the treatment window and show that rt-PA is effective beyond 3 hours. ECASS III will be a double-blind, randomized, placebo-controlled trial in the 3–4 h time window with approximately 400 patients per study arm and the ECASS II dose of rt-PA. The primary endpoint will be a mRS score of 0–1 at day 90, the secondary endpoint will be a global outcome (mRS 0–1, BI 95–100, GOS 0–1) at day 90. Safety parameters will include symptomatic ICH rate, survival at day 90, and also rates of brain herniation and symptomatic brain edema. Inclusion criteria will be age 18–80, clinical diagnosis of stroke (NIHSS score ≤24) without significant improvement, informed consent, treatment possible within 3–4 hours. Exclusion criteria will be similar to ECASS II, including early CT signs of ICH or extensive infarction. Recruitment will start in early 2003.

The benefits of arterial recanalization may be supplemented by neuronal protection (first protocol drafts underway), particularly when the two strategies are used simultaneously, and if they can be used very early following symptom onset. A very interesting approach is the ultrasound-enhanced recanalization under treatment with rt-PA. There are intravascular devices (EKOS, EPAR, Angiojet), but no data are presently available. Clot lysis facilitation with transcranial ultrasound is another option. Two trials are underway: TRUMBI is an international trial, CLOTBUST is an oligocentric trial headed by the University Medical Center at Houston, Texas. Preliminary unpublished data from CLOTBUST (A.V. Alexandrov, J.C. Grotta) showed a significantly higher rate of *early* recanalization in patients treated with rt-PA and ultrasound as opposed to rt-PA alone. Further data are pending.

■ Phase IV Trials of Intravenous Thrombolysis and Cost Aspects

After FDA approval of rt-PA for intravenous thrombolytic therapy in June 1996, the rate of thrombolysis remained fairly constant until the end of 1998 [124]. At most centers where thrombolysis is performed, the NINDS protocol is used; many of these centers also use the ECASS-CT criteria of early infarction. Despite of Level I evidence in favor of thrombolysis, it is estimated that overall only 1% of all ischemic stroke patients and 2% of the time eligible (3 h window) are treated with rt-PA, a rather low rate. This has several reasons such as persisting doubts, fear of hemorrhage, or inadequate reimbursement. The reported outcome and complication rates seem to be similar to the NINDS trial in most instances. The CASES registry in Canada has registered more than 1000 rt-PA-treated patients with a median NIHSS score of 15, a symptomatic ICH rate of 4.6% and a rate of 46% independent patients (mRS 0–2). In Cologne, Germany, approximately 22% of the patients who arrive within 3 hours after symptom onset (5% of all ischemic stroke patients) receive thrombolysis [118]. This rate was achieved after a cooperation between emergency caregivers, internists and neurologists was initiated and the referral system optimized. The average door-to-needle time in Cologne is 48 minutes. The rates of total, symptomatic, and fatal ICH were 11%, 5%, and 1%, respectively. Of these patients, 53% recovered to a fully independent functional state. Recently, the same group published their data on long-term follow-up after thrombolytic therapy, where 150 patients treated within 3 hours were reevaluated after 12 months [310]. After 12 months, 41% of the patients had an MRS score of ≤ 1 and 52% of ≤ 2. The stroke recurrence rate (6.6%/year; TIA 3.3%/year) was consistent with that of population-based studies [293]. These results are nearly identical to the late follow-up outcome analysis published by Kwiatkowski et al. in 1999 [188]. In Houston, 30 patients were treated prospectively after the NINDS protocol [61]. Six percent of all patients hospitalized with ischemic stroke received intravenous t-PA at the university hospital and 1.1% at the community hospitals. The rates of total, symptomatic, and fatal ICH were 10%, 7%, and 3%, and 37% of patients recovered to fully independent function. The average door-to-needle time was 1 hour 40 minutes.

Two very recent studies presented divergent results: Albers et al. reported the STARS (Standard Treatment with Alteplase to Reverse Stroke) study results, a phase IV trial mandated by the Food and Drug Administration [3]. STARS was a prospective, multicenter study of consecutive patients, who received intravenous rt-PA according to NINDS criteria. Outcome measurement was the MRS at 30 days. Here, 389 patients received rt-PA within 2 hours 44 minutes, and the median baseline NIHSS score was 13. The 30-day mortality rate was 13%, 35% of patients had very favorable outcomes (MRS ≤ 1), and 43% were functionally independent (MRS ≤ 2) at day 30. Another 3.3% of the patients experienced symptomatic ICH, which was fatal in 7 patients. Asymptomatic ICH was seen in 8.2%. Protocol violations were reported for 32.6% of the patients and consisted mostly of treatment after 3 hours (13.4%) mainly due to a door-to-needle time of 1 hour 36 minutes, treatment with anticoagulants within 24 hours of tPA administration (9.3%), and tPA

administration despite systolic blood pressure exceeding 185 mmHg (6.7%). The authors conclude that favorable clinical outcomes and low rates of symptomatic ICH can be achieved using tPA for stroke treatment, while the time effort for emergency evaluation may leave room for logistic improvement. Another study by Katzan et al. yielded different results [170]. Twenty-nine hospitals in the metropolitan area of Cleveland, Ohio, prospectively assessed the rate of rt-PA use, rate of ICH, and outcomes in 3948 stroke patients. Seventy patients (1.8%) admitted with ischemic stroke received rt-PA. Sixteen patients (22%) experienced ICH; 11 of these patients (15.7%) had a symptomatic ICH (of which 6 were fatal), and 50% had deviations from national treatment guidelines. In-hospital mortality was significantly higher (P < 0.001) among patients treated with tPA (15.7%) than in patients not receiving rt-PA (5.1%). The fact that blood pressure guidelines were followed in only 47.8% and that the baseline NIHSS score was only documented in 40% of the patients illustrates that intravenous thrombolysis, though an effective therapy, should be performed at experienced centers only and may explain the substantially higher rate of mortality and ICH in this study compared to other investigators. Unpublished data from Canada and Germany and our own data confirm the impression that the efficacy and risk of thrombolytic therapy seen in the controlled trials can be matched or even improved in the clinical setting.

The costs associated with intravenous thrombolytic therapy will be a factor in determining the extent of its utilization. Fagan et al. analyzed data from the NINDS study and the medical literature were used to estimate the health and economic outcomes associated with using tPA in acute stroke patients [87]. A Markov model was developed to compare the costs per 1,000 patients treated with tPA compared with the costs per 1,000 untreated patients. In the NINDS rt-PA Stroke Trial, the average length of stay was significantly shorter in tPA-treated patients than in placebo-treated patients (10.9 versus 12.4 days; P = 0.02) and more tPA patients were discharged to home than to in-patient rehabilitation or a nursing home (48% versus 36%; P = 0.002). The Markov model estimated an increase in hospitalization costs of $1.7 million and a decrease in rehabilitation costs of $1.4 million and nursing home costs of $4.8 million per 1,000 treated patients with a greater than 90% probability of cost savings. The estimated impact on long-term health outcomes was 564 (CI 3 to 850) quality-adjusted life-years saved over 30 years of the model per 1,000 patients, which makes a net cost savings to the health care system likely. With growing experience and better training of emergency medicine personnel, internists, and neurologists throughout all stroke services, the efficacy of intravenous thrombolytic therapy with rt-PA may even improve, and the time window may be routinely extended to 6 hours after symptom onset.

■ Trials of Intraarterial Thrombolysis for Acute Ischemic Stroke

Results of several case series on local thrombolysis in the carotid artery territory have been promising, although not convincing [22, 79, 86, 122, 148, 149, 161, 168, 231, 296, 340, 350, 351, 394, 395]. For rt-PA, doses ranged between 10 and 80 mg; for urokinase, doses usually ranged up to 1.5 million units. Time from symptom onset to treatment in the smaller series has been for the most part within 6 hours, but not within 3 hours or even 4 hours of symptom onset with regard to the mean or median. The reported complete or partial recanalization rates vary substantially between less than 50% [231] and more than 90% [79, 395]. When combining the results of these case series, complete clot lysis is reported for 67 of 174 patients (39%). Partial clot lysis with partial recanalization is reported for 62 of the same 174 patients (36%). The combined partial or complete recanalization rate for these patients was 75%, clearly higher than that demonstrated in the angiography-based intravenous studies (approximately 55%). Each of these intra-arterial case series differs from all of the others with regard to thrombolytic agent, baseline neurological deficit, angiographic anatomy, time-to-treatment, outcome, and method of neurological evaluation at follow-up. Accordingly, con-

clusions regarding efficacy are not possible. The most feared complication of local intra-arterial therapy for stroke, as for intravenous thrombolytic therapy, is ICH. Symptomatic ICH based on the case series is estimated to be 4%, which is lower than that reported for any intravenous thrombolysis series. However, this rate is also lower than that reported in the PROACT I and II trials, in which 24-hour CT scans were performed on all patients. Other complications of intra-arterial thrombolysis include arterial intracranial embolization, subarachnoid hemorrhage, arterial perforation, secondary embolization, hemorrhagic infarction, groin hematoma, and retro-peritoneal hematoma. These complications occur infrequently, certainly in less than 5% for all the series combined. One drawback of intra-arterial in contrast to intravenous thrombolysis is the considerable time delay to angiography, and from initiation of angiography to clot lysis [22, 86, 395]. A recent open study by Arnold et al. evaluated the safety and efficacy of local intra-arterial thrombolysis using urokinase (mean dose 860,000 IU) in patients with acute stroke due to MCA occlusion in 100 patients [7, 112]. The median baseline NIHSS score was 14, angiography showed occlusion of the M1 segment of the MCA in 57 patients, of the M2 segment in 21, and of the M3 or M4 segment in 22, and on average, 236 minutes elapsed from symptom onset to therapy. Of the patients, 47% had an excellent outcome (mRS 0 to 1), 21% a good outcome (mRS 2), and 32% a poor outcome (mRS 3 to 6) with 10% deaths. Recanalization as seen on angiography was complete (TIMI 3) in 20% of patients and partial (TIMI 2) in 56% of patients. Age <60 years (P < 0.05), low NIHSS score at admission (P < 0.00001), and vessel recanalization (P = 0.0004) were independently associated with excellent or good outcome and diabetes with poor outcome (P=0.002). Symptomatic ICH occurred in 7% of the patients. Even if Arnold et al. treated nearly as many patients as were in the treatment arm in PROACT II, their study has an open, non-randomized design which does not suffice for Level I or II recommendations or FDA approval of urokinase.

There are limited data (Phase I and II) only at present to support the combined use of intravenous and intra-arterial thrombolysis with rt-PA. A protocol of the Bridging group uses 0.6 mg/kg with a 10% to 20% bolus and continuous infusion up to a maximum of 60 mg rt-PA [201]; when angiography is started, the infusion is stopped. The rest of the dose up to 90 mg maximum is given intra-arterially. The underlying rationale for this approach is the reduction of any delay for thrombolysis, while still having the higher recanalization rate and proven larger time window for therapy with the intra-arterial approach. Preliminary data in a phase II trial suggest a reasonable safety profile efficacy of this technique [42]. The final data have not been reported in written form yet. It has to be noted that the combination of i.v. and i.a. therapy utilizes the time saving i.v. route and the higher and faster recanalization rates of the i.a. approach. However, this protocol should be limited to clinical investigations and is not based on any study results; thus, it cannot be recommended as a routine procedure.

PROACT I was a randomized phase II trial of recombinant pro-urokinase (rpro-UK) versus placebo in patients with angiographically documented proximal middle cerebral artery occlusion [80]. Angiography was performed after exclusion of ICH by CT. Patients displaying TIMI grade 0 or 1 occlusion of the M1 or M2 middle cerebral artery were randomized 2:1 to receive rpro-UK (6 mg) or placebo over 120 minutes into the proximal thrombus face. Recanalization efficacy was assessed at the end of the 2-hour infusion and symptomatic ICH at 24 hours. A total of 105 patients underwent angiography; 65 of these (N = 25: no occlusion, N = 36: no M1 or M2 occlusion, N = 2: time interval >6 hours, N = 2: complications) were excluded from randomization. Among the 40 treated patients, 26 received rpro-UK and 14 placebo at a median of 5.5 hours from symptom onset. Recanalization was significantly associated with rpro-UK (P = 0.0085) and TIMI 3 recanalization was achieved in 5 rpro-UK patients, as opposed to none of the placebo patients. ICH occurred in 15.4% of the rpro-UK-treated patients and 7.1% of the placebo-treated patients (non-significant); all patients with rpro-UK *and* early CT signs of >33% suffered ICH. In patients who received high-dose adjuvant heparin, the recanalization rate was 81.8%; in the low-dose heparin group (dose was lowered for reasons of safety by the safety committee) it was 40% (P = 0.0255). Mortality was lower in the rpro-UK group, albeit not significantly.

PROACT II, a randomized, controlled, multicenter, open-label clinical trial with blinded follow-up, aimed to determine the clinical efficacy and safety of intra-arterial rproUK in patients with acute stroke of less than 6 hours duration caused by MCA occlusion [102]. Eligible patients had new focal neurological signs attributable to the MCA territory, allowing initiation of treatment within 6 hours after symptom onset, a minimum NIHSS score of 4 points, and exclusion of ICH on CT. Patients with these criteria underwent angiography and were randomized (2:1) to either treatment with 9 mg rpro-UK/2 hours plus the PROACT I lower dose of heparin (2000 IU bolus, 500 IU/hour continuous infusion) or heparin alone. Mechanical disruption of the clot was not permitted. After 1 hour (4.5 mg rpro-UK), a control angiogram was performed and even if the clot had partially or completely dissolved, the rest of the rproUK dose was administered. The primary outcome was the rate of patients with a MRS of ≤2 at 90 days. Secondary outcomes included MCA recanalization (TIMI 2 and 3), the frequency of symptomatic ICH, and mortality. Of 12,323 patients screened in 54 centers, only 474 (4%) underwent angiography at a median of 4.5 hours after stroke onset, 294 of which demonstrated angiographic exclusion criteria, leaving 121 rpro-UK and 59 control patients with a median baseline NIHSS score of 17 points for ITT analysis. Further, 40% of rpro-UK patients and 25% of control patients had a MRS of 2 or less (absolute benefit 15%, relative benefit 58%, number needed to treat = 7; P = 0.04). Mortality was 25% for the r-proUK group and 27% for the control group (P = 0.8). The recanalization rate was 66% for the r-proUK group and 18% for the control group (P < 0.001); TIMI 3 recanalization rates were 19% and 2%, respectively (P < 0.003). All other secondary outcomes were nonsignificant. Early ICH occurred in 35% versus 13% of patients (P = 0.003); at 10 days the rates were 68% and 57% (P = 0.23). Early symptomatic ICH occurred only in patients with NIHSS scores >11 within 24 hours in 10.2% of r-proUK patients and 2% of control patients (number needed to harm = 12; P = 0.06). The results of PROACT II did not suffice for FDA approval. Another study of intra-arterial pro-urokinase for acute stroke within 6 hours (PROACT III) is planned but due to funding problems still a matter of debate.

In summary intra-arterial thrombolytic therapy of acute M1 and M2 occlusion with 9 mg/2 hours significantly improves outcome if administered within 6 hours after stroke onset. Seven patients need to be treated in order to prevent one patient from death or dependence. The higher rate of symptomatic ICH (10.2% in PROACT II versus 8.8% in ECASS II, 6.4% in NINDS and 7.2% in ATLANTIS) is very well explained by the far larger baseline severity of stroke in PROACT II (NIHSS score of 17 in PROACT II versus 11 in ECASS II and ATLANTIS, and 14 in NINDS). According to the Cochrane meta-analysis [379, 380], combining PROACT I and II data (34), there is a 0.55 OR (CI 0.31–1.00) for death or disability, an OR of 2.39 (CI 0.88–6.47) for early symptomatic ICH (7 to 10 days), and an OR of 0.75 (CI 0.4–1.42) for death from all causes at follow-up. Although recanalization rates may be superior with intra-arterial (66%) than with intravenous (≈ 55%) thrombolysis and may even be increased by careful mechanical disruption of a thrombus, in addition to the lytic effect of the drug, a limited availability of centers with 24 hour a day – 7 days a week interventional neuroradiology service may restrict the use of this therapy. On the other hand, the clinically more severe strokes may benefit even more from an intra-arterial than an intravenous approach. Furthermore, the time to eventual recanalization may be substantially shorter with intra-arterial thrombolysis.

Thrombolytic Therapy for Vertebrobasilar Infarction

Vertebral basilar distribution cerebral infarction has been of particular interest to centers experienced with local intra-arterial thrombolysis. Six large case series [27, 40, 47, 100, 133, 395] have been published since 1986. The early and first series by Hacke et al. [133] retrospectively investigated the clinical-angiologic data and the clinical outcome in 66 patients with angiographically demonstrated thrombotic vertebrobasilar artery occlusions who received either local intra-arterial thrombolytic therapy (urokinase or streptokinase) (43 patients) or conventional therapy (antiplatelet agents or anticoagulants) (22 patients). Recanalization in patients who received thrombolytic therapy correlated significantly with clinical outcome; in 19 of 43 patients, recanalization was demonstrated angiographically, while in 24 patients the occlusion persisted. All patients without recanalization died, but 14 of the 19 patients displaying recanalization survived (P = 0.000007), 10 with a favorable clinical outcome. Only three of the 22 patients who received conventional therapy survived, all with a moderate clinical deficit. When we compared the treatment groups, highly significant differences in both outcome quality (P = 0.017) and survival (P = 0.0005) were found to depend on establishing recanalization. These data support the concept that technically successful thrombolysis of vertebrobasilar artery occlusions is associated with beneficial clinical outcome. The great majority of the more than 120 patients (from all studies) treated were administered intra-arterial urokinase locally; a few patients were given rt-PA. Treatment was almost always delayed such that no patients were reported in these series as having been treated within 3 hours of symptom onset. The median time from the beginning of treatment to the time of recanalization was reported to be 120 minutes [395]. For the total group, the complete or partial recanalization rate is approximately 70%; in reality the rate probably is somewhat lower, as partial or complete recanalization is usually not achieved in 100% of patients, as reported by Zeumer et al. [395]. Mortality of vertebrobasilar thromboembolism is high, with overall rates of approximately 70–80%. Successful recanalization, however, was associated with a survival rate of 55% to 75%, as opposed to 0–10% in persistent or untreated basilar artery occlusion [40, 133]. Two thirds of the survivors after recanalization had a favorable outcome; all survivors in the untreated group were moderately disabled. Other authors reported an overall mortality of 75% in 13 patients; although ten of these had experienced recanalization [27], non-recanalization led to death in all patients (N = 3). The authors concluded that recanalization of the vertebrobasilar system is necessary but not sufficient for effective treatment of vertebrobasilar occlusive disease [27]. To address the potential risks and potential benefits of intra-arterial thrombolysis for vertebral basilar artery occlusion more fully, a randomized trial (The Australian Urokinase Stroke Trial) is planned but has not been started to date because of expected low recruitment numbers [76]. Grond et al. reported one small case series of 12 consecutive patients in whom they investigated whether early intravenous thrombolysis could also effectively be applied in acute vertebrobasilar ischemic stroke [117]. Patients with clinically diagnosed moderate to severe vertebrobasilar ischemic stroke with clearly determined symptom onset were treated with intravenous rt-PA within 3 hours after symptom onset, following a protocol similar to that of the NINDS study. On admission, 7 patients exhibited moderate to severe brainstem symptoms without impairment of consciousness and 5 patients had impairment of consciousness, of whom 2 were comatose. Of 12 patients, 10 had a favorable outcome after 3 months, defined as full independence (Barthel index score of 100) or return to premorbid condition. One patient had a poor outcome with complete dependence due to reocclusion after primarily successful thrombolysis, and one patient died of severe brainstem infarction and additional space-occupying parietal hemorrhage. Unfortunately, basilar artery occlusion was not demonstrated by any means, such as Doppler ultrasound, CT or MR angiography, or digital subtraction angiography. The utility of Doppler ultrasound and CTA in the diagnosis of vertebrobasilar occlusion, however, has been studied and demonstrated by Brandt et al. [38] who showed a greater than 90% sensitivity and specificity for CTA but only 30% for Doppler ultrasound. In four patients with acute basilar artery thrombosis, complete arterial recanalization

and good neurologic outcome were achieved with a treatment combining alteplase with tirofiban, a glycoprotein IIb/IIIa inhibitor with lytic capacity for platelet thrombi [167]. In no cases were cerebral or extracerebral hemorrhagic complications observed.

In summary, the natural disease course of vertebrobasilar occlusion has a grim prognosis. Neuroradiological intervention with intra-arterial thrombolysis to date is the only life-saving therapy that has demonstrated benefit with regard to mortality and outcome, albeit not in a randomized trial. However, sufficient data are available to justify intra-arterial thrombolytic therapy in the light of mortality and disability in these patients. The time window for thrombolysis in the posterior circulation has not been established but may be up to and even exceed 12 hours, although Fox et al. suggest a time window of more than 10 hours to be associated with a poor prognosis [100]. Presence or absence of vertebrobasilar vessel occlusion can be safely, noninvasively, and rapidly established by CT (or MR) angiography before a neuroradiological intervention is initiated. The data for intravenous thrombolysis in vertebrobasilar obstruction are too scarce for any recommendation to be made, but warrant further study.

■ Recommendations for Thrombolysis

Overall, thrombolysis with 0.9 mg/kg rt-PA for acute ischemic stroke within 6 hours leads to a clinically significant effect in favor of treated patients but is associated with an excess rate of symptomatic ICH, which does, however, not take effect on mortality. Intravenous rt-PA (0.9 mg/kg; maximum of 90 mg) is therefore the recommended treatment within 3 hours after stroke symptom onset. Thrombolytic therapy should be performed in centers experienced with the procedure. The benefit from the use of intravenous rt-PA for acute ischemic stroke beyond 3 hours from onset of symptoms is lower, but definitely present in selected patients. Also, the European Stroke Initiative (EUSI) recommendations state that thrombolytic therapy is the therapy of choice within 3 hours and in selected patients up to 6 hours after stroke onset [334]. The adjunctive use (and also the optimal timepoint of use) of antithrombotic agents is still controversial and at present no recommendation can be given with regard to concomitant administration of heparin or antiplatelet agents in the setting of thrombolytic therapy. Intravenous rt-PA is not recommended when the time of onset of stroke cannot be ascertained reliably; this includes patients in whom strokes are recognized upon awakening. Intravenous administration of streptokinase for acute ischemic stroke is dangerous and contraindicated. Data on the efficacy of any other intravenously administered thrombolytic drugs are not available such that a recommendation could be provided. Intra-arterial thrombolysis with recombinant pro-urokinase is safe and effective within 6 hours after stroke onset, leading to a significantly higher rate of functional independence, also in patients with more severe baseline stroke symptoms. For vertebrobasilar artery thrombosis, intra-arterial thrombolysis, although not proven in randomized trials, if successful, may dramatically reduce mortality and disability, and therefore is the therapy of choice within 6 but eventually up to 12 hours after symptom onset. Improvements in early diagnostic evaluation of patients, particularly in MRI techniques, allow a better patient selection and possibly a qualification of the presently rigid therapeutic time frame.

Intravenous rt-PA has been approved with restrictions for stroke patients in Germany since August 2000 and without restrictions since 2001 in South America. The mutual recognition procedure, however, did not result in a Europe-wide approval of rt-PA. Finally, approval for rt-PA within 3 h has been given Europe-wide after an arbitration procedure, where evidence and expert reports have been reviewed and reevaluated. Preliminary restrictions for patients older than 75 years or with regular pre-stroke use of platelet inhibitors were not based on any data and thus are not understood by these authors. However, they have been amended in the revised version of the approval. Furthermore, in analogy to the CASES registry, a European rt-PA for ischemic stroke registry called SITS-MOST where every patient treated with rt-PA within 3 hours has to be reported to will be compulsory. SITS-MOST is internet based and will be located in Stockholm.

However, at present thrombolytic therapy is still underutilized. Among the major problems are that relatively few candidates meet the clinical and time criteria. Educating the general public to regard stroke as a treatable emergency and training emergency caregivers in the use of thrombolysis may decrease these problems. Healthcare institutions should be made aware of the potential in long-term cost savings, once stroke management is optimized and thrombolysis is more widely available. Patients and their relatives should be informed not only about the hazards of thrombolytic therapy but also about its potential benefit and thus the risk of *not* being treated.

12 Impact of Stroke MRI on Therapeutic Decision Making

P. D. Schellinger, J. B. Fiebach, S. Warach, W. Hacke

Intravenous thrombolysis with rt-PA is effective in acute stroke patients [304, 305]. Although tPA is the only proven therapy for acute stroke, only 3% to 4% of all stroke patients are currently treated [251]. The limited use of rt-PA is partly due to safety concerns of neurologists, internal medicine and emergency physicians [21, 170] and the narrow therapeutic time window. The extension of the therapeutic window would be an important step towards a broader application. It has been argued that the selection of stroke patients likely to respond to thrombolysis might improve functional outcome within the 3 h time window and extend the window towards 6 hours after stroke onset [2, 131]. In this chapter we discuss, how stroke MRI can be used to guide acute therapy especially whether to give or withhold thrombolytic therapy. In essence, the presence of a vessel occlusion according to MRA is associated with a PWI/DWI-mismatch, the stroke MRI setting that defines the ideal candidate for thrombolysis [281, 307]. In addition, early recanalization achieved by thrombolysis results in significantly smaller infarcts and a significantly better clinical outcome [160, 173, 213, 302, 307]. Detection of old as well as new microbleeds and early hemorrhagic infarction by T2*-WI may allow the exclusion of patients from thrombolysis, who have an excessive bleeding risk [172, 175, 246]. This association, however, has to be firmly established first. Also patients with biphasic infarctions may be identified.

A prospective, open-label, non-randomized multicenter trial (five university hospitals) examined the MRI baseline characteristics of patients with acute ischemic stroke and studied the influence of intravenous rt-PA on MR parameters and functional outcome in 139 patients (76 rt-PA versus 63 controls) within

6 h after symptom onset and on follow-up [288]. The objectives were to define the prevalence and size of mismatch and lesion volumes in acute stroke patients, to assess the effect of rt-PA on recanalization rates, whether time point of thrombolysis and recanalization rate do have an impact on functional outcome and whether the vascular occlusion pattern is associated with mismatch volume and functional outcome. All patients were studied within a multiparametric stroke MRI protocol within 6 hours after symptom onset and for follow-up. The NIHSS (baseline) and mRS (day 90) scores were assigned by experienced local stroke neurologists. Patients were divided into two therapeutic groups: the no-thrombolysis group with conservative treatment and the thrombolysis group with thrombolytic therapy. Conservative treatment was defined as thrombocyte aggregation inhibitor and low molecular weight heparin s.c. as a prophylactic measure for deep venous thrombosis. Baseline characteristics, lesion volumes, mismatch ratio, occlusion types, recanalization, and functional outcome were compared between groups. All patients eligible for thrombolysis received a CT study either before or immediately after the MRI protocol to exclude intracerebral hemorrhage. Stroke MRI was performed before thrombolysis (n=63) or immediately after application of rt-PA (n=10; median 65 minutes, range 12–120 min). MRI follow-up was performed at days 1 and 7. Recanalization was assessed from the follow-up MRI study on day 1 on the basis of the PWI and MRA studies according to the modified Thrombolysis in Myocardial Infarction (TIMI) criteria [339]. The two groups did not differ concerning age and sex, however, the initial NIHSS was lower (P=0.002) and time to MR was longer (P=0.002) in the no-thrombolysis group. Five

patients had symptomatic intracerebral hemorrhage (2 with and 3 without thrombolysis). Ten patients died within the follow-up period of 90 days (4 with and 6 without thrombolysis). Median time to thrombolysis was 180 minutes (45–333 min). Forty-five patients were treated within the 3 h time window and 31 within the 3–6 h time window. MRI was performed 180 min (75–360 min) after the start of symptoms. A relevant mismatch (mismatch ratio >1.2) was present in 120 of 139 patients (86.3%). MRA demonstrated a vessel occlusion in 90% of patients. The mismatch ratio did not differ (P=0.39), whereas the mismatch volume was smaller in the no-thrombolysis group (P=0.032). Mismatch ratio and mismatch volume did not differ within the subgroups of patients treated within the 3 h and 3–6 h time window (mismatch ratio, P=0.75; mismatch volume P=0.69). The final lesion volume (T2-WI on day 7) was smaller in the thrombolysis group with 35 ml (1.6–377 ml) vs. 73 ml (0–685 ml): p=0.079.

Of the 19 patients without a mismatch (mismatch ratio <1.2), 8 (42%) had no vessel occlusion on MRA as compared to 6 from 120 patients (5%) in the group with a mismatch. Two characteristic patterns were identified: a) eight patients without mismatch, but patent vessels and normal PWI, had small average initial DWI lesion volumes of 3 ml (1–43 ml) and final infarct volumes of 10 ml (0–54 ml), less severe initial NIH stroke scores with a median of 10 (1–17 ml) and good functional outcomes (mRS ≤2: 87.5%). b) Eight patients with average initial DWI lesion volumes greater than 70 ml (mean 174 ml, range 73–254 ml) had large final infarct volumes (mean 194 ml, range 17–421 ml), high initial NIHSS scores (median 17, range 7–20) and a poor clinical outcome (mRS ≥3 in 5/8 patients: 62.5%). Data on vessel recanalization were available in 125 of 139 patients (90%). Dichotomized TIMI criteria for TIMI 0–1 (no recanalization or minimal recanalization) and TIMI 2–3 (recanalization with residual perfusion deficit and complete recanalization) showed a trend towards an effect of rt-PA in the thrombolysis group (TIMI 2–3: 32.4% vs. 21.2%; P=0.22). Dichotomizing TIMI 0 versus TIMI 1–3 showed a stronger effect of rt-PA on recanalization rates (P<0.001). In 45 pa-

tients (59.2%), thrombolysis was performed within 3 hours whereas 31 patients (40.8%) were treated in the 3–6 h time window. We did not find an effect of early (≤3 h) versus late (3–6 h) thrombolytic therapy on the mRS (dichotomized RS ≤2 vs. 3–6: P=0.48). Dichotomizing patients for RS ≤1 vs. 2–6 had no effect (P=0.49). Patients treated within the 3-hour time window showed higher recanalization rates than the 3–6 h group (TIMI 1–3: P=0.024). Recanalization had an effect on the mRS: 67.6% patients with TIMI 2–3 had a good outcome (RS$_{90}$≤2) as compared to 42.7% of patients with TIMI 0–1: P=0.016; dichotomization RS ≤1 vs. 2–6: P=0.001). Dichotomization in TIMI 0 (33.9%) versus TIMI 1–3 (64.1%: P=0.001) showed a comparable effect. Multiple logistic regression analysis was performed to detect simultaneous influences on the functional outcome (dichotomized mRS ≤2). Age, thrombolytic therapy within 3 hours, T2 lesion volume day 7, and the initial NIHSS score had a significant effect on the outcome. Thrombolytic therapy within 3–6 hours showed a trend towards a better outcome that was not as strong as tPA therapy within 3 hours (3 hour group OR 0.14 vs. 3–6 hour group OR 0.35). Dichotomizing mRS ≤1 vs. 2–6 resulted in a significant effect of thrombolysis in the 3–6 h time window (P=0.02). No effect was seen for the mismatch ratio, mismatch volume, initial DWI and PWI volumes, recanalization rate, time of thrombolytic therapy and the occlusion type (Figs. 12.1 and 12.2).

In summary, the findings of Röther et al. are that patients most likely to achieve neurologic independence (mRS 0–2) were younger, had milder baseline stroke severity (NIHSS score) and were treated with rt-PA. This rt-PA benefit was achieved, although the initial NIHSS score was higher in the thrombolysis group. Interestingly, the beneficial effect of rt-PA was independent from the 3 h or 3–6 h time window, although thrombolysis in the 3 h time window appeared more effective than in the 3–6 h time window. One might hypothesize that a reasonable explanation for worse outcomes within a delayed time window might be smaller volumes of tissue-at-risk-of-infarction, worse initial NIHSS score, larger DWI volumes to start with or larger fi-

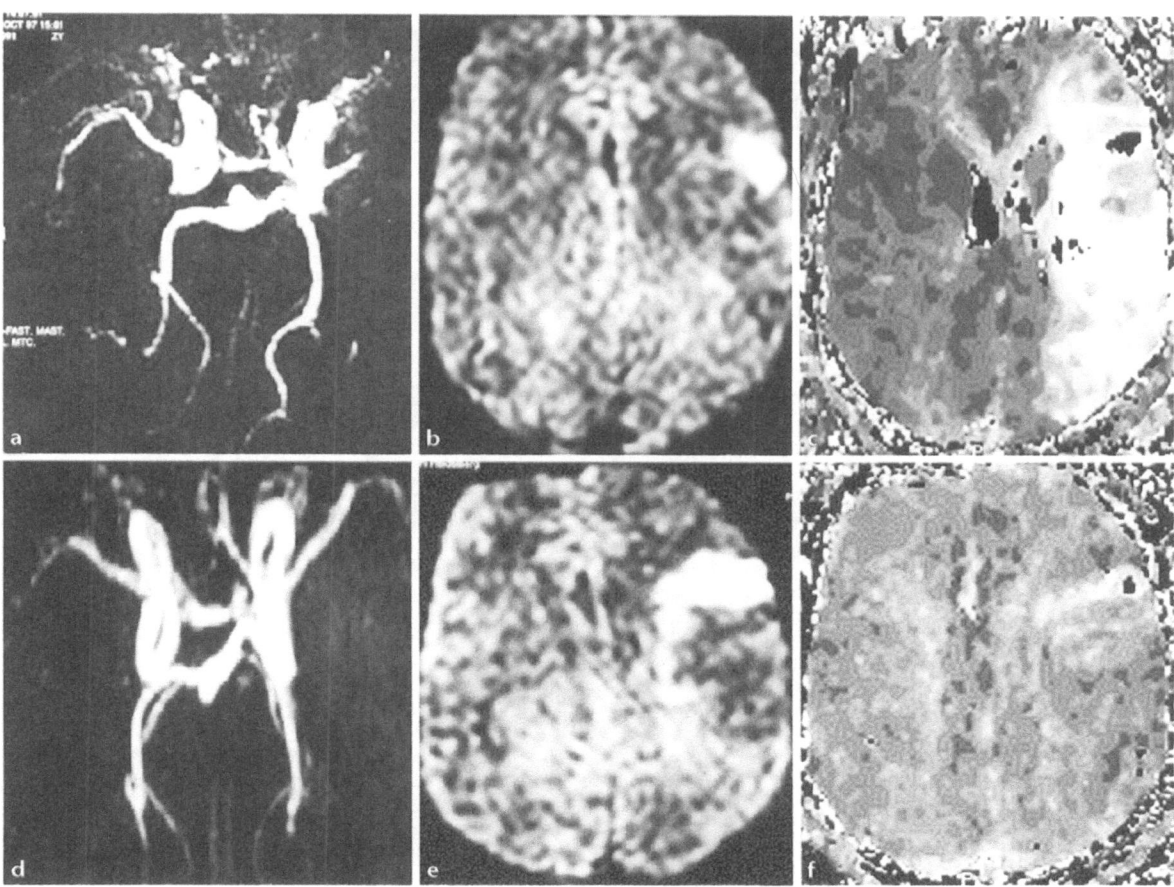

Fig. 12.1. The initial CT findings (1 h after symptom onset) in this 46-year-old patient were normal. Stroke MRI was performed 2 h 30 min after symptom onset. The initial stroke MRI (**a–c**) shows from left to right a proximal MCA occlusion on MRA, a small, left cortical, hyperintense lesion on DWI and a hypoperfusion of the complete left MCA territory on PWI (large PWI/DWI-mismatch). After thrombolysis (**d–f**), the infarction has not significantly increased according to DWI (**e**) but perfusion has returned to normal except for a small left frontal deficit in the ischemic core (**f**); MRA reveals that the MCA has recanalized (**d**). The patient initially presented with a NIHSS score of 14; after successful thrombolysis his day 90 exam resulted in a NIHSS of 1, BI of 100, and mRS of 1

nal infarct volumes. However, Röther et al. did not find differences within the subgroups in the 3 h and 3–6 h time window as far as these parameters are concerned. They therefore conclude that MRI has the potential to become a valuable tool to select patients likely to benefit from thrombolysis beyond a rigid time window based on their individual time window. It is obvious that nutritional reperfusion is likely to contribute to smaller final infarct volumes and favorable outcome. Since thrombolytic therapy favored recanalization, it is further likely that the beneficial effect of thrombolysis on functional outcome is mediated by higher recanalization rates and smaller lesion volume.

It is a topic of ongoing discussions whether lacunar stroke patients or patients with spontaneous recanalization might benefit from thrombolysis. Some authors argue that, based on the assumption that rt-PA has its effects through recanalization of larger angiographically visible arteries or that outcome is related to recanalization anyway (none of the large trials assessed recanalization), rt-PA should not be withheld in patients with small vessel disease [225]. Also, the authors of NINDS state that lacunar strokes in their trial profited as well as large vessel or embolic strokes. However, their diagnosis of lacunar stroke was not based on imaging but a clinical assumption and, thus, in our opinion is not val-

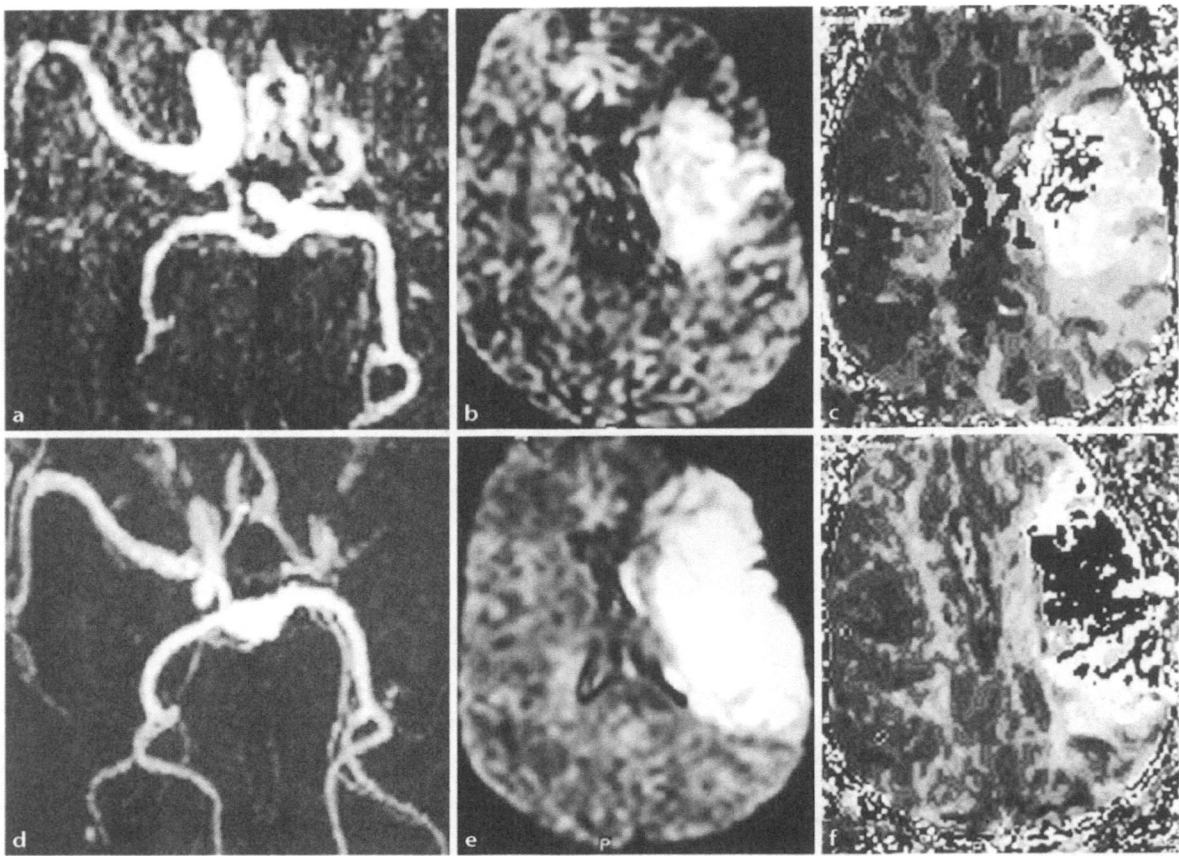

Fig. 12.2. This 49-year-old patient had an unremarkable initial CT (1 h after symptom onset) except for an early hyperdense sign of the left MCA. On the initial stroke MRI (**a–c**) (1 h 15 min after symptom onset), the left insular cortex and putamen are hyperintense (**b**). PWI shows hyperintensity of most of the left MCA territory, reflecting a marked hypoperfusion (**c**) and a large PWI/DWI-mismatch. MRA shows a proximal left-sided distal internal carotid and M1 occlusion (**a**). After thrombolysis (**d–f**), the patient's status did not improve. Follow-up DWI shows a large MCA infarction (**e**) with persistent perfusion deficit, according to PWI (**f**), and a persistent vessel occlusion on MRA (**d**). The patient had a poor outcome with a BI of 55, and a mRS of 4 at day 90

id. One might expand these arguments and ask whether thrombolysis should be limited to patients with DWI/PWI-mismatch. As the rationale for thrombolytic therapy is the lysis of an obliterating thrombus with restoration of blood flow and salvage of hypoperfused tissue at risk of infarction as identified by stroke MRI, we do not generally recommend rt-PA in these patients (Fig. 12.3).

Stroke physicians are frequently confronted with stroke patients, in whom the exact time of symptom onset is not known, e.g., who have a deficit when awakening [96], or the patient is not in the condition to give the required information due to aphasia or disorientation. At present, patients like these are excluded from thrombolytic therapy even if a CT scan does not demonstrate any or only minor ischemic changes. Accordingly thrombolysis as an effective therapy may be withheld from patients who might profit from rapid recanalization. Therefore, we suggest that patients presenting with symptoms of acute stroke of unknown onset time and without CT-contraindications for rt-PA should be investigated with stroke MRI and should be given thrombolytic therapy if a vessel occlusion and a substantial mismatch are present, possibly even when only a perfusion deficit is present and a very cautiously phrased informed consent can be obtained by the patient or his/her closest relatives.

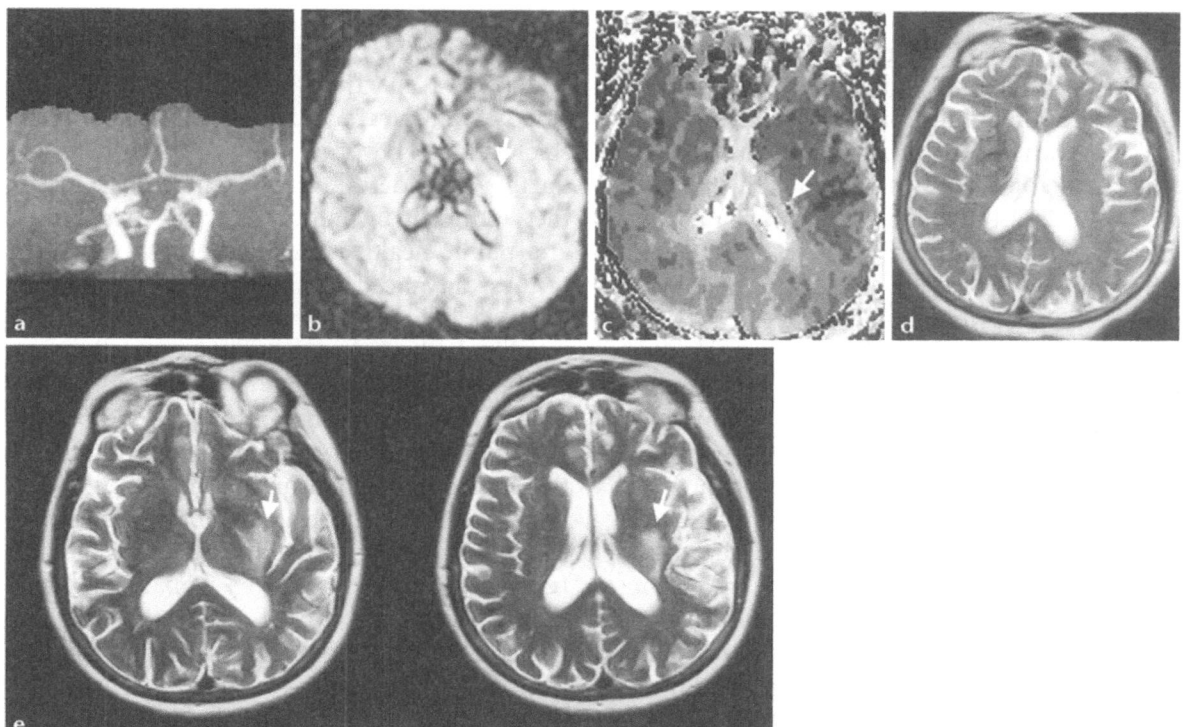

Fig. 12.3. This 73-year-old patient experienced an acute severe right-sided hemiparesis, hemihypesthesia, facial palsy and dysarthria (NIHSS score 11). The initial CT 3 h 40 min after symptom onset was normal; stroke MRI was performed within 4 hours after symptom onset. MRA (**a**) and T2-WI (**d**) are normal, on DWI (**b**, *arrow*) there is a lacunar infarction on the left side in the internal capsule and, on PWI (**c**) there is a small corresponding area of hypoperfusion (3 voxels). The patient's symptoms improved spontaneously and she was without any symptoms on day 90 (mRS 0). The follow-up T2-WI (**e**) demonstrate the lacunar infarct (*arrows*)

There are no data presently available that sufficiently document the utility of imaging techniques for decision making in vertebrobasilar stroke. CTA has been shown to be significantly superior to DU in demonstrating basilar artery occlusion [38, 39]. Stroke MRI has been used in our center as an exclusion criterion for neuroradiological intervention when large brainstem, bithalamic and bilateral PCA infarctions could be demonstrated. However, sensitivity of DWI and especially PWI at the base of the skull is low due to bone-associated susceptibility artifacts. Neuroradiological intervention with intra-arterial thrombolysis to date is the only life-saving therapy that has demonstrated benefit with regard to mortality and outcome, albeit not in a randomized trial. However, sufficient data are available to justify intra-arterial thrombolytic therapy in the light of mortality and disability in these patients. The time window for thrombolysis in the posterior circulation has not been established but may be up to and even exceed 12 hours, although Fox et al. suggest a time window of more than 10 hours to be associated with a poor prognosis [100].

We are aware that our recommendations are not based on a randomized, controlled double blind trial and do not meet the criteria of an officially approved therapy. However, as there is already a substantial and still growing body of evidence in favor of the recommended procedures, these recommendations may be seen as an expert consensus and provide the rationale for an individual therapeutic approach in an institutional protocol. The fact that an individual therapy based on advanced knowledge is offered, which does not meet the criteria of drug approval institutions and therefore may be associated with a higher risk of hazardous if not fatal side effects, must be stressed when informed consent is obtained. Conversely, it should be stated that the drawback of a later onset of therapy may be outweighed by a sophisticated diagnostic imaging procedure telling the physician whether to treat or not to treat. Patients and their relatives should be informed not only about the hazards of thrombolytic therapy within or outside the 3 h time window but also about its potential benefit and thus the risk of *not* being treated.

In summary we hypothesize that the optimal comprehensive diagnostic workup of acute stroke patients should not be limited to non-contrast CT as a means of excluding ICH, even if this is the present standard and absolute minimum procedure in the 3 h time window. It can safely be assumed that a sophisticated differential indication for thrombolysis requires information about the presence or absence of a vessel occlusion whether by means of DU, CTA, or MRA in the 3 h and should be obtained in the 3–6 h time window. While optional but nevertheless optimal for patients within the 3 h time window, advanced information such as clear demarcation of the irreversibly damaged infarct core and the ischemic but still viable thus salvageable tissue at risk of infarction as seen on DWI/PWI/MRA should also be obtained before thrombolysis is initiated within 3–6 h. There is no evidence available showing that patients without demonstration of an occlusion and with a PWI/DWI-match (e. g., lacunar stroke) might not profit from therapy. While this does not seem likely to these authors, one might consider giving therapy in individual cases applying the view in terms of there being neither a relevant indication nor a contraindication and thus proceed with treatment. A mismatch without vessel occlusion is a hypothetical constellation but may be seen in distal MCA branch occlusions, where the occlusion may not be detected by rapid MRA sequences. Due to the presently still low but increasing availability of stroke MRI as opposed to a wide distribution of modern CT scanners, a CT/CTA/CTA–SI protocol with or without DU is the diagnostic alternative in these instances. However, it has to be reiterated that randomized prospective and blinded trials to back these rationally well-based hypotheses are still lacking and should be the

next step (such as the EPITHET and DEFUSE trials currently being employed in Australia and USA, respectively). Therefore we call for a large randomized, controlled trial utilizing stroke MRI beyond the 3 h time window. Further considerations are time constraints in the setting of thrombolysis, cost effectiveness and public health issues as well as availability of these advanced technologies. These authors, however, believe that the latter obstacles can be or already have been at least partially overcome.

We suggest that there are four distinct categories of patients: in one of these (number 2) the indication for thrombolysis in our opinion is moderate at best and not based on evidence but on questionable pathophysiological reasoning and thus may be a matter of individual debate; in two of these, thrombolytic therapy should also be an urgent consideration in the 3–6 h time window and in infarctions of less than 33% of the MCA territory according to DWI:

1) We recommend to abstain from thrombolysis in patients with large infarctions exceeding 50% of the MCA territory according to DWI,

2) The indication for intravenous thrombolysis is a matter of debate but not performed at our center in a) patients without PWI/DWI-mismatch but with vessel occlusion, b) patients with PWI/DWI-mismatch but without (identifiable) vessel occlusion (e. g., distal MCA branch), c) without proof of vessel occlusion and without mismatch (e. g., lacunar stroke), d) individual patients with PWI/DWI-mismatch, vessel occlusion and DWI lesion volume between 33% and 50% of the MCA territory,

3) i.v. and/or i.a. thrombolysis are indicated and essential in patients with MCA occlusions distal to the lenticulostriate branches and with presence of a PWI/DWI, and

4) Recanalization should be achieved by all means in patients with distal ICA or proximal MCA occlusions and presence of a PWI/DWI-mismatch.

As an alternative to CTA or MRA, DU may be employed, if the time constraints in the setting of thrombolytic therapy can be met. Comprehensive informed consent is mandatory, especially when thrombolytic therapy is considered beyond established time windows.

With regard to the controversially discussed utility of stroke MRI due to its low availability [267, 268, 397], we believe that the constellation of the DWI, PWI, MRA, T2-WI and PWI/DWI-mismatch allows the early identification of those patients in whom outcome and final infarct size, ultimately the patient's fate, have not yet been determined. With an increasing distribution and 24 h/d and 7 d/week availability of stroke MRI, the identification of patients suitable for thrombolytic therapy, and those who are not, will lead to an increased benefit and a reduction of complications [307]. Furthermore, the rather strictly defined therapeutic window may be qualified and individualized according to the findings in each patient.

13 Alternative and Future Imaging Prospects

P. D. Schellinger, J. B. Fiebach, K. Sartor

■ Doppler/Duplex Ultrasound

The most widely available tool to non-invasively assess extracranial and intracranial vessel status is Doppler/duplex ultrasound [25] which is a suitable bedside tool not only for baseline vessel status but also to monitor the process or absence of recanalization, whether rt-PA is applied or not. Already early DU-reports described that rapid recanalization is associated with a higher rate of clinical improvement and smaller infarcts at outcome [277]. Clinical recovery from stroke correlates with the timing of arterial recanalization after thrombolysis, complete recanalization was common in patients who had follow-up Rankin Scores of 0 to 1 (P = 0.006) [62]. rt-PA results in a faster recanalization, significantly higher recanalization rate (66% versus 15% in controls), and therefore in a significantly smaller infarct volume and a significantly better clinical outcome at 3 months [5, 227]. Secondary ICH, which is associated with a worse clinical outcome, is significantly more frequent in patients with late rather than early recanalization [228]. A pilot multicenter study evaluated color-coded duplex sonography in acute stroke patients before and after rt-PA therapy [104]. Recanalization of the occluded MCA after 2 and 24 h was diagnosed in 50% and 78% of the patients treated with rt-PA and in 0% and 8% in the control group. This is in accordance with data from MRI studies [302] and illustrates that the largest effect of thrombolytic therapy is seen, when rt-PA is given to patients, in whom a vessel occlusion has been established. A potential disadvantage of DU, however, is its examiner-dependent sensitivity, sensitivity for branch occlusions and time consumption as well as potential problems with uncooperative patients and lack of a transcranial insonation window.

■ CT/CTA/CTA Source Images (CTA-SI)

CT angiography (CTA) by using spiral CT today is a widely available tool to evaluate the circle of Willis. In acute ischemic stroke patients, this technique can provide accurate information on stenoses or occlusions in the basal arteries of the brain [178, 319]. Direct comparison of CTA and DU suggests that the results from CTA compare favorably with ultrasound and that CTA can also reliably detect intracranial stenosis, emboli and aneurysms of a moderate or larger size [206]. The method is non-invasive, safe and independent from the grade of experience of the investigator (in contrast to Doppler sonography). In a large series of stroke patients none had any immediate adverse reactions after administration of the intravenous nonionic iodinated contrast material [319]. Newer generations of CT scanners allow for lower contrast doses. While older studies reported an increase of the infarct size after administration of ionic contrast material, an experimental study clearly showed that bolus injection of nonionic contrast material does not affect infarct volume or worsen the symptoms of cerebral ischemia [82], although this should be more firmly established. CTA is superior to Doppler sonography in the assessment of basilar artery patency in patients with the syndrome of an acute basilar artery ischemia, particularly in patients with distal basilar artery occlusion (Fig. 13.1) [38].

In addition to the assessment of a major vessel occlusion, CTA has the potential to deliver information about the quality of the collateral circulation. In patients with good leptomeningeal collaterals, contrast enhancement in the arterial branches beyond the occlusion occurs. This degree of enhancement can be taken as an estimate of the collateral blood

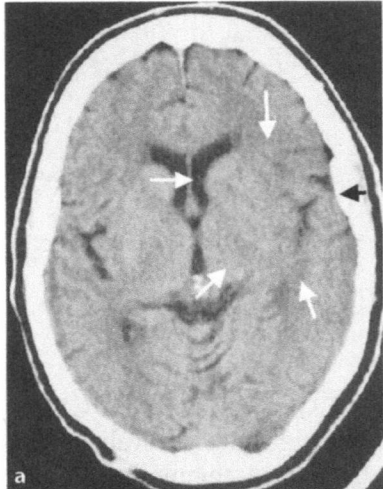

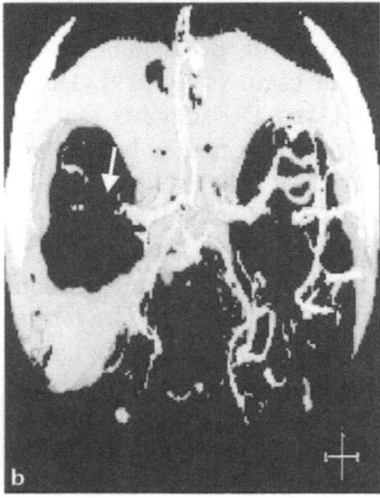

Fig. 13.1. a CT of a patient with sudden onset of a right-sided hemiparesis and aphasia. The non-contrast CT shows early signs of infarction, e.g., loss of the insular ribbon, sulcal effacement and hypoattenuation of the lentiform nucleus (*arrows*). **b** CTA demonstrates a proximal MCA occlusion on the left (*arrow*)

flow [177, 389]. However, CTA may have limitations such as being less reliable in showing branch occlusions of the middle cerebral artery or other smaller vessels distal to the circle of Willis [177, 319]. On the other hand, it can easily be performed directly after non-contrast CT. A standard CTA protocol may be as follows: 65 ml of a nonionic contrast medium are injected into a cubital vein at a rate of 5 ml/s using an injection pump. After a delay of 15–20 seconds, spiral scanning is performed with a slice thickness of 2.0 mm, an index of 1.5 mm, and a spiral pitch of 1.25 at

130 kV and 125 mA. For diagnosis, the CTA-SI and the 3-dimensional reconstruction of the data sets can be used.

In addition to the vessel status, CTA-SI may provide indirect information about the collateral circulation and may also improve the contrast of perfused and malperfused brain areas, thus, increasing the sensitivity for early ischemic changes not seen on non-contrast scans [178, 199, 389]. Analysis of CTA-SI must be clearly differentiated from perfusion CT, where analogous to perfusion-weighted MRI (PWI), a contrast bolus tracking method is applied and hemodynamic parameters may be assessed [181]. CTA-SI analysis is a stronger predictor of clinical outcome than the initial NIHSS score and may predict final infarct volume and clinical outcome. Patients with recanalization do not experience infarct growth, whereas those without complete recanalization do [200]. While stroke MRI is the new gold standard in stroke imaging, these techniques are not widely available yet. Modern CT scanners on the other hand are more widely available and less expensive than MRI scanners; they are often located in the emergency departments even of smaller community hospitals. Acute stroke is not only treated at specialized academic medical centers; indeed, the majority of patients present first in local general hospitals that have no MRI facilities [141]. Schramm et al. therefore investigated whether CTA-SI allows detection of ischemic brain lesions in patients with acute ischemic stroke, whether their sensitivity is comparable to that of DWI, whether the hypoperfused brain area seen on CTA-SI correlates with the final infarct and whether the qualitatively assessed collateral status reflects the risk of infarct growth [311]. The clinical and imaging findings of 20 consecutive stroke patients (7 women, 13 men; mean age 61±10 years) imaged within 6 hours (45 min to 5 h 45 min) after stroke onset with both imaging modalities were analyzed. CT was performed within the first 45 min to 4 h 45 min after stroke onset (mean 2.83 h±1.33 h), followed by MRI (range from 1 h 15 min to 5 h 30 min after symptom onset; mean 3.38 h±1.37 h). The time interval between CT and MRI ranged from 15 min to 1 h (0.55 h±0.25 h). Of the 20 patients, 16 had a vessel occlusion seen on both CTA and MRA. All but one of these 16 patients had an abnormal initial DWI scan. Five of these patients showed good collaterals, and 11 showed poor collaterals surrounding the lesion site. All vessel occlusions detected on CTA were seen on MRA at the same location. In every patient, the status of the collateral vessels surrounding the lesion was determined on the CTA-SI; seven patients showed good intravascular enhancement of the perilesional vessels and were classified as "good", 13 patients showed only poor enhancement around the lesion site and were classified as "poor". Neither in patients with poor collaterals (P=0.807) nor in patients with good collaterals (P=0.6) did CTA-SI lesion volumes differ significantly from DWI lesion volumes (P=0.601) at baseline. In patients with poor collateral vessel status, initial CTA-SI lesion volumes differed significantly from T2-WI lesion volumes on day 5 (P=0.0058), whereas in patients with good collaterals no significant difference was found (P=0.176). Day 1 DWI lesion volumes differed significantly from T2-WI lesion volumes on day 5 in patients with poor collaterals (P=0.0035), respectively, whereas in patients with good collaterals the difference did not reach statistical significance (P=0.176) signaling profound lesion growth in patients with poor collateral status. In all patients, the lesion volume measured in CTA-SI significantly correlated with the initial lesion volumes on DWI (P<0.0001, r=0.922) and with the outcome lesion volume on day 5 T2-WI (P=0.013, r=0.736). Furthermore, patients with good collaterals uniformly had a significantly better clinical outcome on day 90 as measured by four neurological and outcome scales (NIHSS: 0±0 vs. 10±7; SSS: 58±0 vs. 35±15; BI: 100±0 vs. 45±45; mRS: 0±0 vs. 4±1; all P≤0.012). For two dichotomized clinical outcomes (mRS 0–1 vs. 2–6: good vs. bad; mRS 0–2 vs. 3–6: independent vs. dependent or dead), a poor col-

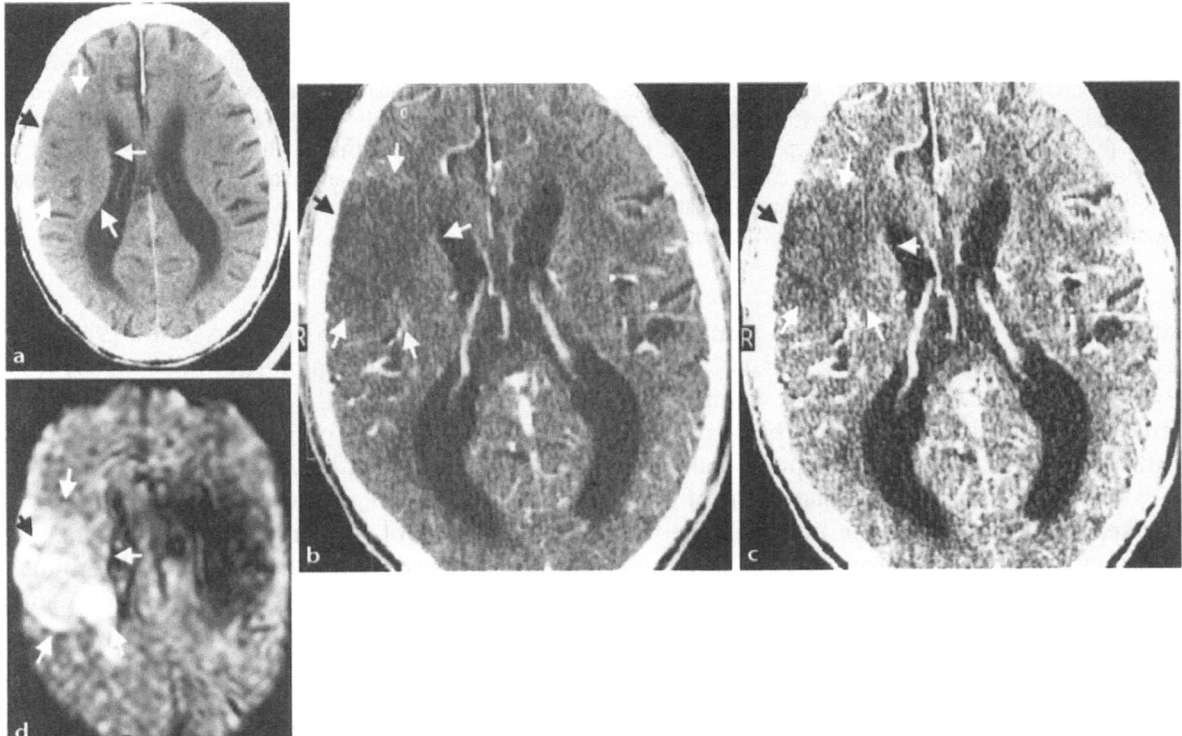

Fig. 13.2. Improved sensitivity with CTA source image analysis. The non-contrast CT (**a**) shows a subtle right frontal hypodensity and sulcal effacement (*arrows*). CTA source images (**b** middle, and **c** right) depict the lesion with a higher sensitivity due to hypocontrastation of the infarct core (*arrows*). Here it is evident that window and level settings have to be optimized to obtain a good black/white contrast (**c**). On CTA-SI, the lesion (*arrows*) corresponds well to the findings on DWI (**d**)

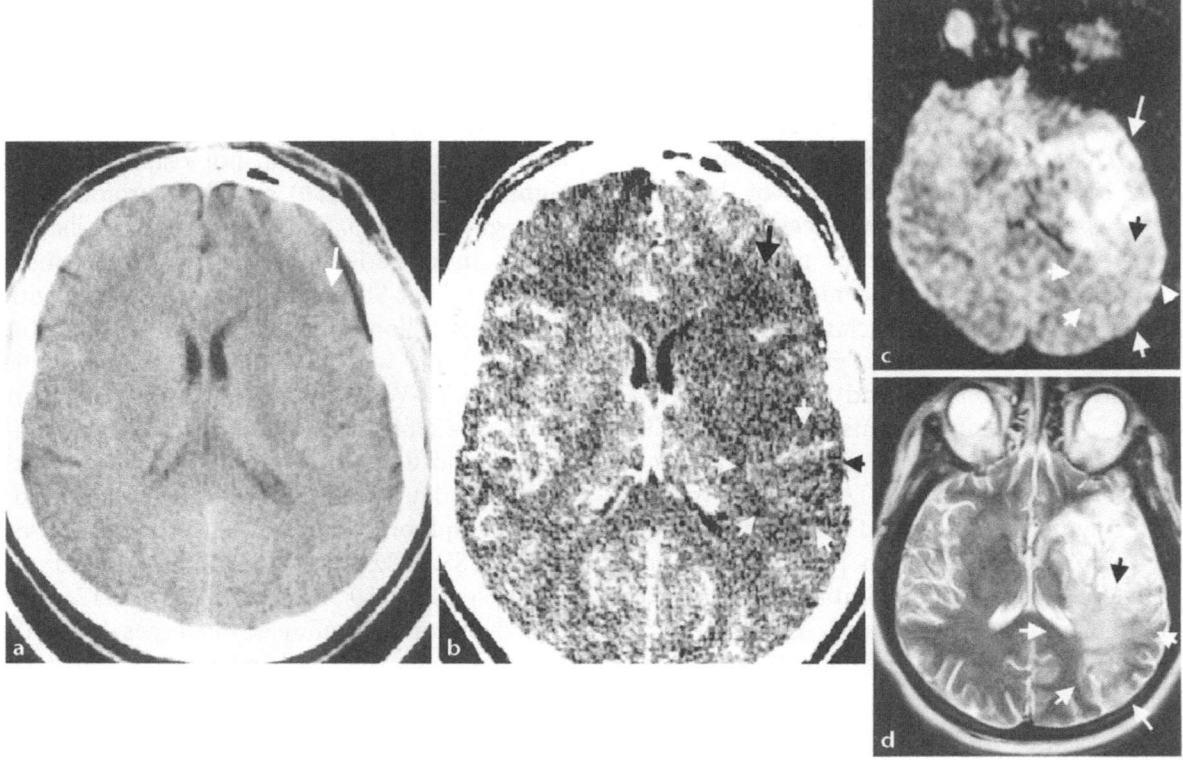

Fig. 13.3. CTA-SI illustrating a mismatch. The non-contrast CT (**a**) shows a mild hypodensity in the frontal cortex (*arrow*) *but does not demonstrate the extent of the infarction.* CTA-SI (**b**) show an area of profound hypodensity due to a complete lack of contrast filling (*single arrow*), the infarct core. Dorsal to the infarct core, there is an area that is not hypodense but only shows a rarefication of leptomeningeal vessels signaling a poor collateral status (*arrows*). On DWI (**c**), this area is not infarcted yet (*small arrows*) as opposed to the infarct core (*single arrow*). T2-WI (**d**) on follow-up show that due to failing collaterals the tissue at risk depicted by CTA-SI did not recover and proceeded to irreversible infarction (*arrows*)

lateral status also predicted a significantly worse clinical outcome (P = 0.025 and P = 0.001). Day 5 T2-WI lesion volumes differed between the subgroups, being significantly larger in patients with poor collaterals (P = 0.024). Thus, in the management of acute stroke, when stroke MRI is not available, the decision to initiate thrombolytic treatment should be based on the clinical findings and CT scanning including CTA (Figs. 13.2 and 13.3).

The reported diagnostic yield of non-contrast-enhanced CT within 3 h after symptom onset is low [70, 126, 322]. On the other hand, detection of X-ray hypoattenuation on CT is highly specific for irreversible brain damage, also within the first 6 hours after ischemic stroke. Still, the sensitivity in diagnosing ischemic stroke is substantially lower than on DWI in the first few hours [94]. CTA can increase the diagnostic value of CT [38, 178, 199, 389]. As the substrate for thrombolytic therapy is an obliterating thromboembolus, the ability of CTA to detect intracranial vessel occlusion suggests that it is a useful screening tool for identifying patients in whom intravenous or intraarterial thrombolysis is appropriate [229]. Since the therapeutic time window for thrombolytic therapy is only 3 hours and up to 6 hours in selected patients, the need for an improved, CT-based diagnostic tool is evident. A normal non-contrast-enhanced CT scan in acute stroke does not imply insensitivity of the method; in fact, it represents the favorable situation in which ischemic edema has not yet developed and the chance to avoid irreversible damage is still good. Unenhanced CT does not show the arterial occlusion itself; it even does not show the extent of disturbed cerebral perfusion. One might ask if standard post-contrast CT should not suffice to visualize the extent of ischemic tissue. However, in comparison to post-contrast CT, CTA has the advantage of showing the leptomeningeal collaterals surrounding the lesion of reduced parenchymal enhancement which can be seen with both methods. In patients with a poor collateral vessel status, CTA-SI may provide information similar to that of the PWI/DWI-mismatch concept, analogous to the findings of Jansen et al. and Schellinger et al. [160, 302]. The volume of the affected brain area that has an inadequate blood supply can be estimated by the difference between the CTA-SI lesion volumes and the brain area supplied by the occluded artery, taking the qualitative assessment of the collateral status into account. The patients with poor collaterals seem to represent those that may have a PWI/DWI-mismatch, analogous to stroke MRI, and the patients with good collaterals those patients without tissue at risk (i.e., small stroke, lacunar stroke, or tissue at risk already completely infarcted). The combination of CT and CTA may also be more cost effective than stroke MRI. However, the problem in managing acute stroke imaging is not deciding between CT or MRI since the majority of acute stroke patients are admitted to hospitals without MR scanners. Regarding secondary prevention (e.g., antithrombotic treatment), even today many stroke patients do not receive appropriate medication because of lacking brain-imaging facilities, or receive antithrombotic treatment without a prior CT scan to exclude intracranial hemorrhage, also representing an increased risk for those patients [60, 155]. Considering this fact, the combination of CT and CTA is very effective and efficient. Further studies should examine the value of the combination of CT/CTA/PCT in comparison to DWI/PWI MRI. A prospective multicenter trial for acquiring data in a substantially larger set of hyperacute stroke patients is underway.

■ Dynamic Perfusion CT

Whereas CTA and CTA-SI solely provide angiographic information about the circle of Willis and collateral vessels, perfusion CT provides information about the cerebral blood flow (CBF). However, the necessary perfusion software is not yet available on many CT scanners serving emergency units. Dynamic CT during first pass of a bolus of iodinated contrast agent by unidirectional X-ray tube rotation results in images that can be used to generate functional maps of cerebral blood volume (CBV), cerebral blood flow (CBF) or time-to-peak enhancement (TTP). These functional maps of PCT enable the stroke physician to assess cerebrovascular parameters and their changes in acute stroke patients [138, 139]. Areas with reduced CBF can be shown immediately after vessel occlusion with high contrast to areas with normal perfusion. In a recently published study by Koenig et al., perfusion CT was performed within 6 hours of symptom onset in 32 patients with acute stroke symptoms. Comparison with SPECT, performed immediately after perfusion CT, and follow-up CT showed a good correspondence in 81% of the patients [181]. In another study by the same author the findings on different functional maps of cerebral perfusion CT in stroke patients were compared with early ischemic changes on conventional CT [180]. The baseline CT scans of 45 acute stroke patients were retrospectively evaluated with respect to early CT findings. For each patient the extent of cerebral ischemia as shown on the maps of CBF, CBV, and TTP was compared and the severity of ischemia was assigned to one of three levels based on the findings of the CBF image. In 75% of these patients conventional CT was performed within 2 hours from symptom onset. Of 45 patients, 29 showed early signs of ischemia on conventional CT, whereas perfusion CT revealed cerebral ischemia in all patients. Severe ischemia was found in approximately the same rate of incidence in patients with early CT changes (55.2%) and in those with normal findings (43.8%). If the perfusion impairment was judged as mild or moderate the extent of the hypoperfused area was significantly larger on the CBF and TP images than on the CBV map. This was significantly different in patients with severe hypoperfusion where a complete correspondence of the affected area between the three functional maps was found. The authors concluded that the use of conventional CT for the assessment of stroke in the hyperacute phase is limited and that PCT yields excellent information regarding the severity and extent of ischemia. In addition, the use of various perfusion maps may help to differentiate the core of infarction from the ischemic penumbra zone. Besides the delineation of hypoperfused brain tissue, the characterization of ischemia with respect to severity is of major clinical relevance, because the degree of hypoperfusion is the most critical factor in determining whether an ischemic lesion turns into an infarct or returns to normal brain tissue. In another study, Koenig et al. aimed to determine whether measurements of the relative CBF, relative CBV, and relative TTP can be used to differentiate areas undergoing infarction from reversible ischemic tissue [182]. In 34 patients with acute hemispheric ischemic stroke <6 hours after onset, PCT was used to calculate rCBF, rCBV, and rTTP values from areas of ischemic cortical and subcortical gray matter. Results were obtained separately from areas of infarction and noninfarction, according to the findings on follow-up imaging studies. The efficiency of

each parameter to predict tissue outcome was tested. There was a significant difference between infarct and peri-infarct tissue for both rCBF and rCBV but not for rTTP. Threshold values of 0.48 and 0.60 for rCBF and rCBV, respectively, were found to discriminate best between areas of infarction and noninfarction, with the efficiency of the rCBV being slightly superior to that of rCBF. The prediction of tissue outcome could not be increased by using a combination of various perfusion parameters. Thus, the assessment of cerebral ischemia by means of perfusion parameters derived from perfusion CT provides valuable information to predict tissue outcome. In some patients, the ischemia was located outside the scanning level of perfusion CT and was therefore missed. This demonstrates one disadvantage of the method, because with each bolus injection only one brain section (multislice CT a maximum of two 1-cm slices) can be evaluated. However, in some of the patients of Koenig et al. ischemia was located outside the scanning level of perfusion CT and was therefore missed. It is possible to obtain a second bolus injection to perform another perfusion CT, however, it is impossible to evaluate the total brain (Fig. 13.4).

Röther et al. investigated 22 patients within 143±96 minutes of stroke onset with CTP and CT within the first 6 hours of symptom onset

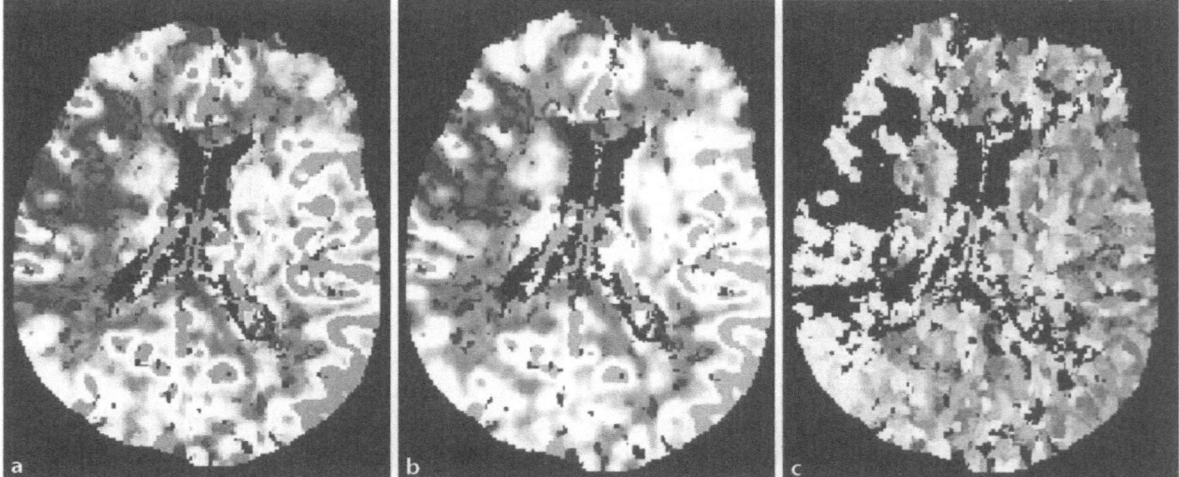

Fig. 13.4. Perfusion CT maps: **a** rCBF, **b** rrCBV and **c** rMTT. There is an area of hypoperfusion in the right MCA territory corresponding to a distal MCA mainstem occlusion seen as hypointensity on the rCBF and rrCBV maps and as hyperintensity on the rMTT maps. These images look similar to perfusion maps from stroke MRI. The validity of this information, especially with regard to rCBF and rrCBV maps still has to be established

and before the start of treatment in a consecutive clinical series. The area of the perfusion deficit from TTP maps, hemispheric lesion area from follow-up CT, final infarct volume, and stroke recovery (NIHSS-score) was assessed. Eighteen patients had perfusion deficits in the middle cerebral artery territory and corresponding hypoattenuation in follow-up CT. Three patients with normal CTP findings showed lacunar infarctions or normal findings on follow-up CT. In one patient, CTP did not reveal a territorial deficit above the imaging slice. The overall sensitivity and specificity of CTP for the detection of perfusion deficits in patients with proven territorial infarction (n = 18) on follow-up CT were 95% and 100%, respectively. New and already available developments in CT technology, including dynamic scanning with multisection data acquisition (multislice CT), may further increase the value of this technique and provide information about the three-dimensional extent of cerebral ischemia. Electron beam computed tomography is also capable to perform multislice dynamic CT with calculation of absolute CBV and CBF. In a small series of 11 patients with acute stroke symptoms, this technique demonstrated reduced CBV and CBF in the 4 patients with proven infarcts on follow-up CT. Disadvantages were caused by high image noise, limiting the demarcation of ischemic tissue [50]. All the general problems with absolute quantitative CBF measurements for DSC MRI also hold true for PCT (see chapter 6).

MR Spectroscopy

Like DWI and PWI proton MR spectroscopy provides information about metabolic changes that may occur before the onset of tissue changes evident on CT scans or T2-weighted MR images. Various metabolite signals may be detected in a proton MR spectrum, including lactate, an indicator of ischemia in the acute phase of stroke, and N-acetyl-aspartate (NAA), believed to be a neuronal marker. In animal experiments increased lactate was detected in the central ischemic region within 1.3 hours after the onset of permanent occlusion. After 1 hour of temporary focal ischemia, lactate returned to nearly normal levels within 0.4 hour after the onset of reperfusion, suggesting that lactate is a sensitive early marker of ischemia but does not predict irreversible damaged tissue [151]. MR quantification of NAA as the neuronal marker during acute ischemia reflects primarily changes of the intracellular NAA [294]. It is suspected that NAA depletion within the early stroke period identifies the central ischemic region that is destined for infarction. The combination of lactate and NAA can therefore perhaps be used to identify with MR spectroscopy the infarct core and a tissue at risk, making MR spectroscopy a useful diagnostic tool for use in the evaluation of acute stroke. The earlier studies of proton MR spectroscopy in human stroke used single-voxel localization techniques [49]. Using this methodology, it has been found that elevated lactate and decreased NAA levels can be detected in stroke patients comparable to experimental findings. Single-voxel techniques, however, do not provide information regarding the spatial distribution and extent of metabolic abnormalities, and require that the location of the ischemic or infarcted region be already known or visible on MR images. There have, therefore, been successful efforts to develop spectroscopic imaging methods for the study of cerebral ischemia. In small recently published series, it could be shown that spectroscopy imaging is feasible for imaging patients with acute stroke and more studies are currently underway to prove whether this technique can identify tissue at risk or even the penumbra [105]. Besides the development of 2- or even 3-dimensional spectroscopic imaging, the development of phosphorus spectroscopic imaging is being pursued, knowing that the measurement of a phosphorus metabolite gives more detailed views of the energy store than a proton metabolite. Full slice spectroscopic imaging at 3 T may also be a suitable tool to track pharmacological substances, e.g., for neuroprotectants whether they topographically reach the brain area they are supposed to have an effect on.

PET and SPECT

The uptake of the tracer HMPAO in the brain tissue is proportional to the actual cerebral blood flow. For this reason HMPAO is regarded as a perfusion-reflecting tracer and HMPAO-SPECT can be used in acute cerebral ischemia to detect areas of abnormal perfusion. The focal absence of HMPAO is a hallmark of arterial occlusion. This information can be acquired within an imaging time of 20 minutes, but an additional time of 30 to 60 minutes is necessary for preparation of the tracer. Images can be interpreted on a visual or semiquantitative basis using a region-to-cerebellar ratio or asymmetry index, but no quantitative data on CBV or CBF can be obtained with SPECT. However, one investigator showed that patients with an extensive deep ischemia on HMPAO-SPECT have a high risk of secondary hemorrhage if local intra-arterial thrombolysis is performed [349]. SPECT with HMPAO can be interesting in prospective clinical treatment studies, because the tracer remains trapped in the tissue, allowing reproducible imaging during the first 4 hours because of minimal washout from the brain. Therefore, a study design with application of the tracer prior to treatment and a secondary SPECT-imaging is possible without a large time delay [6].

PET is the only validated method to measure the absolute CBV or CBF. Using quantitative multitracer PET studies it is possible to visualize the irreversibly damaged tissue, the penumbra and also the area of oligemia in an acute ischemic stroke patient. However, absolute quantitation of the CBF requires knowledge of the arterial input function, which can only be obtained by continuous arterial blood sampling during the PET study. This requires placement of arterial lines, which is contraindicated in patients who may be potential candidates for thrombolytic therapy. Moreover, quantitative PET-studies require very complex logistics, which is usually not possible for an around-the-clock service. In addition, in case of an acute interventional treatment, quantitative PET will consume unacceptable time. All these arguments stand for the problems associated with integration of PET into an aggressive treatment concept of acute ischemic stroke. Since quantitative measures of CBF could not be obtained in acute stroke patients, Heiss and colleagues [147] used the relative regional tracer uptake of (^{15}O)-H_2O to estimate the level of residual blood flow in the affected hemisphere. In 12 patients they demonstrated that this technique can semiquantitatively demonstrate critically hypoperfused tissue, which can be preserved from infarction by early reperfusion. However, as with stroke MRI, this technique can not *directly* delineate the penumbra but can only demonstrate a tissue at risk.

While SPECT and especially PET may provide semiquantitative and quantitative hemodynamic data [33, 147], these modalities are not widely available and are, thus, of academic interest. They probably will not have any practical implications for the general stroke patient in the close future.

14 The Role of Stroke MRI in Clinical Trials

S. WARACH, P. D. SCHELLINGER

The disappointingly slow progress in developing effective therapies for ischemic stroke along with the clinical development of diffusion and perfusion MRI has led to a reevaluation of the strategies for the design of stroke clinical trials. Stroke MRI has been proposed and begun to be used in stroke trials as a means of optimizing patient selection and as a direct measure of the effect of treatments on cerebral infarction, as the marker of therapeutic response. The first and only success in developing an approved therapy for acute stroke culminated in the pivotal trials of intravenous rt-PA [338] reported in 1995 and leading to regulatory approval in 1996. The key insight of the designers of these trials was optimizing the sample with regard to time to treatment, requiring patients to be treated within three hours from onset of symptoms. They recognized that very early stroke treatment would be more effective and that the earliest cases are most likely to still have the causative arterial occlusions, which may spontaneously lyse at later times. Thus, patients were included across the broad range of clinical features, and selection of patients by imaging confirmation of the diagnosis or pathologic features most amenable to the treatment was not necessary to prove the efficacy of intravenous rt-PA for the less than three hours time window. In the subsequent six years, many unsuccessful clinical trials for acute stroke have been reported and drug development for many once-promising agents has been abandoned. In particular, trials of intravenous rt-PA initiated up to six hours from symptom onset have failed to demonstrate efficacy in a sample of acute stroke patients selected without imaging confirmation of the diagnosis [70, 125, 126] even if meta-analyses of all these studies suggest efficacy beyond the 3 hour time window [124, 379].

Except for the trials of intravenous rt-PA in the treatment of ischemic stroke within the first three hours, this traditional approach has lead to no approved therapies for stroke and a great degree of pessimism with regard to thrombolysis beyond 3 hours and to the general concept of neuroprotection in stroke. To demonstrate efficacy in a clinical trial with a treatment time window beyond three hours, other features of trial design need to be optimized, and proof of pharmacological activity in Phase II is needed before lengthy, expensive, labor intensive and potentially risky Phase III clinical trials are undertaken. The requirement of proof of concept Phase II studies will prevent the wastefulness of Phase III trials that are doomed to futility before they begin. Image-guided Phase II studies may answer the question of target biological activity in fewer than 200 patients, the sample size typical for Phase II trials. Trends toward benefit using clinical scales at Phase II have been notoriously poor predictors of clinical outcomes in Phase III trials on much larger samples.

It would be unthinkable for clinical trials in cardiology or oncology to enroll patients by bedside clinical impression alone, without objective evidence from diagnostic testing confirming the pathology before inclusion of a patient. Yet this has been the traditional standard by which clinical trials for ischemic stroke have been conducted, because until recently there had been no practical alternative. Rapid MRI diffusion, perfusion, angiography and gradient echo imaging provides that alternative. In using MRI as a selection criterion, the goal would be a sample selection based upon a positive imaging diagnosis of a pathology rationally linked to the drug's mechanisms of action. Requiring a positive diagnosis of acute ischemic injury by DWI and PWI would ideally assure that no patients with diagnoses mimicking stroke are included in the sample, a desirable objective unachievable in trials using bedside impression and non-hemorrhagic CT as the basis of inclusion. The goal of image-based patient selection is to narrow the range of patient characteristics, leading to a more homogeneous sample, reducing within group variance, and increasing the statistical power (lowering sample size requirement) of the experimental design to demonstrate efficacy. The principle of optimal patient selection by imaging confirmation of the relevant pathology was first demonstrated by the results of the intra-arterial pro-urokinase stroke study, PROACT II [102]. In PROACT II 180 patients were selected based on evidence of arterial occlusions at the M1 or M2 levels of the middle cerebral artery by conventional arteriography, and a significant clinical benefit was observed when thrombolysis was initiated up to 6 hours from symptom onset. The results of that trial suggested that a more prolonged study duration, increased expense and potential delay in treatment to complete a screening test may be justified by the greater chance of demonstrating clinical benefit by using a pathologically homogeneous and rational selection of patients. A recent report of a pilot clinical trial of intravenous rt-PA between 3 and 6 hours from onset demonstrated in a subgroup of sixteen patients with diffusion-perfusion mismatch a significant degree of recanalization, reperfusion, and tissue salvage as well as a clinical benefit relative to untreated historical controls as did another multicenter trial comparing stroke MRI features of rt-PA-treated patients (N = 76) with controls (63) in 139 patient all of whom were imaged within 6 hours [258, 288]. These sample sizes are an order of magnitude smaller than was required to show clinical benefits in the rt-PA trials, which did not select a homogeneous sample of patients on the basis of imaging pathology, and supports the concept that selection of an optimal sample may lead to smaller sample size requirements even for clinical endpoints. Optimal patient selection would be based on a positive imaging evidence of the ischemic pathology that the therapy has been developed to treat. The simplest use as an inclu-

sion criterion would include the presence of a lesion on DWI to increase the diagnostic certainty of ischemic stroke. For reperfusion therapies, the optimal target of therapy would be patients with evidence of an arterial occlusion or hypoperfusion with the greatest territory at risk for infarction, i.e., the diffusion-perfusion mismatch [213, 307, 373].

For neuroprotective drugs acting only in cortical areas of ischemic penumbra, optimal selection of patients would be acute lesions involving the cerebral cortex. For some neuroprotective drugs the diffusion-perfusion mismatch may be the optimal target, for other agents that would protect against reperfusion injury or would not achieve sufficient concentration in oligemic tissue, the optimal target would be patients in whom reperfusion has occurred. Patients might also be excluded from the trial at screening if subacute or chronic lesions are found that may confound measurements of lesion volumes or clinical severity as outcome variables. Because of a relative large error of measurement associated with small lesions [193], lesions larger than a minimum volume, e.g., 5 ml, may be desirable. Furthermore, an upper limit of lesion volume at enrollment would permit an opportunity for lesion growth and may better differentiate the effect on lesion size of an effective treatment from placebo. Selection of patients by DWI is also optimally suited for using change in lesion volume as a direct measure of the neuroprotective effect of the drug (Tables 14.1 and 14.2).

Before an experimental stroke therapy is brought from the laboratory to clinical trial,

Table 14.1. Uses of stroke MRI (DWI, PWI, MRA) as a selection tool in stroke trials

Positive radiological diagnosis of ischemic stroke
Select by location appropriate to the therapeutic mechanism
Select by size
For reperfusion therapies select by presence of perfusion defect or by PWI/DWI-mismatch
For neuroprotective drugs select by PWI/DWI-mismatch or reperfusion depending on drug mechanism
Exclude if confounding subacute or chronic lesions

Table 14.2. MRI as outcome measure in neuroprotectant trials

Necessary but not sufficient evidence of protective effect
Protective effect may be attenuation of expected lesion growth or partial DWI lesion reversal
Clinical benefit unlikely if no protective effect on lesion volume (go/no go decision at phase II)
Smaller sample size requirements than for typical clinical endpoints ($\sim$50–100 per arm)
May be confirmatory evidence supporting positive clinical endpoint trial for regulatory approval

it is necessary to demonstrate that the treatment causes reduction in lesion volume in experimental models. The fundamental premise of drug discovery and development in acute stroke is that treatments that reduce lesion size are those most likely to lead to clinical benefit. In clinical trial programs that depend solely on clinical endpoints as indices of benefit, drugs may be brought to Phase III testing without the requirement of evidence that the drug will have the therapeutic effect observed in the experimental model. In practice, this traditional approach to stroke trials has been unsuccessful and often misleading. Four major factors are hypothesized to predict tissue response and clinical efficacy in stroke trials: time to treatment, the salvageable tissue-at-risk, the relevance of the patient sample to the treatment, and the intrinsic effectiveness of the therapeutic strategy [370]. Time is an important factor [214], but it is not the only important factor hypothesized to affect response to therapy. The amount of ischemically threatened and clinically symptomatic but potentially salvageable tissue-at-risk at the initiation of therapy is another factor that is likely to predict clinical response. The ideal sample in a clinical trial should also be treatment congruent. A treatment-congruent sample is a sample comprised of patients most likely to respond to therapy, patients who have the pathology that the therapy is intended to treat, e.g., an arterial occlusion for a thrombolytic trial, and who have other features predictive of a measurable response to therapy. The ideal treatment-congruent sample will also have no features predictive of

serious adverse events. The fourth major factor is the intrinsic effectiveness of a therapeutic approach. Observations in experimental models suggest that reperfusion or neuroprotection by endogenous, pharmacological, or physical mechanisms reduce infarct volume, that reperfusion has a greater benefit on infarct reduction than neuroprotection and that the effect of a combination of reperfusion and neuroprotection is yet greater. The relative effectiveness of a therapy depends not only on its pharmacological properties, but also on choices made in trial design, such as the dosing and method of administration.

The clinical trial optimized on all features would have the most robust response. When the trial is completely optimized on these factors, the pretreatment lesion on DWI is partially reversible. As the factors are progressively less optimized, the lesions are more likely to grow relative to the pretreatment volume and the differences among the types of treatment will progressively decrease to zero. Optimized on one feature, differences in trial efficacy will depend on the value of the other factors. A less effective therapy studied under optimized conditions may show greater efficacy in trials than a truly more effective one, if the latter is studied without optimizing the design along the other dimensions. For example, a later treatment window may nonetheless lead to a positive trial result if the trial design is optimized for efficacy on the other factors, despite lack of efficacy at those times on an indiscriminately selected sample.

Figure 14.1 illustrates the hypothesized relationship of these factors to efficacy in stroke trials using lesion growth on MRI as the marker of therapeutic response. As discussed above, optimizing sample selection may lead to smaller sample sizes, but the greatest advantage for increased power of stroke MRI is the measurement of the pretreatment lesion against which to compare the final lesion. Such an approach to within subject variance must, by basic statistical principles, be more powerful than analysis of only the final lesion volume. The question of whether a treatment causes reduction of lesion volume may be answerable in the study of one to two hundred patients in Phase II, whereas five to ten times as many patients

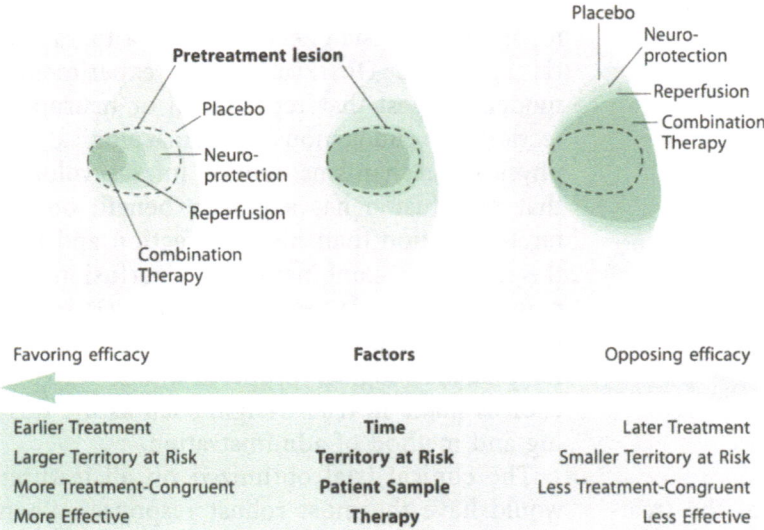

Fig. 14.1. Model of lesion responses in stroke clinical trials: a multifactorial continuum. Illustrated are the principles hypothesized to affect tissue outcome in clinical trials, and the likelihood of demonstrating efficacy on either infarct volume or clinical variables. The three slices depict three points along the hypothetical continuum of tissue response in stroke trials according to the major factors (*center column*) that are hypothesized to affect efficacy. The dashed ovals outline the pretreatment volume of tissue injury on DWI. The solid gray regions depict the final infarct volume as a function of treatment. The change in lesion volume from pretreatment volume is the MRI marker of therapeutic response. The un-treated (placebo) patient will have an amount of lesion growth that is independent of factors affecting efficacy. Reperfusion therapy will have a greater lesion effect than neuroprotective therapy, and the combination of reperfusion and neuroprotection will be best. Trials optimized for efficacy have the features in the left column; trial characteristics that oppose efficacy for each factor are listed in the column on the right. The relative value along each of these dimensions in a clinical trial will interact to determine efficacy on infarct volume as well as clinical outcome. The factors are discussed in the text

are typically tested in Phase III studies in order to evaluate the treatment with clinical endpoints. Thus, a Phase II MRI endpoint trial to replicate the preclinical experiment in a patient population may be a rational and cost effective basis of deciding whether or not to proceed with Phase III testing. A positive lesion outcome study in late Phase II would be supportive of the decision to proceed with Phase III trials. The citicoline MRI trials demonstrated this principle and also substantiated the claim that sample size requirements for an effect on lesion volume may be on the order of 50 to 100 patients when pre-post lesion difference is used as the outcome variable. In the first citicoline MRI trial [377], no significant difference was found on pre-post percentage change in lesion volume between active and placebo, but from that study it was estimated 58 patients per treatment arm would have been required to achieve signifi-cance. In the next citicoline MRI trial using a higher dose, a significant effect of treatment for pre-post lesion volume change was observed in 71 placebo- and 62 citicoline-treated patients, using the baseline NIHSS as a covariate in the analysis [378]. By contrast, in that trial there were no differences in the final infarct size when pretreatment lesion volume assessment was not used, despite a sample size five times as great (337 placebo and 336 citicoline treated). The first citicoline MRI trial [377] also confirmed observations from single center natural history observations that the lesion volumes were significantly correlated with scores on clinical scales, and that the clinical severity (by baseline NIHSS) and the severity of the hemodynamic abnormality (volume of abnormality of PWI) were independent predictors of lesion growth. While other authors have published conflicting data [302], they studied another

patient clientele with substantially more severe stroke patients part of these having been
treated with thrombolytic therapy. The citicoline data, however, suggest the value of PWI
lesion volume and NIHSS score as covariates
of lesion growth in subsequent trials. Reducing the disabling sensory motor, and cogni-
tive deficits associated with cerebral infarction is the clinical goal of acute stroke thera-
peutics, therefore, reduction of infarct volume
is the biological objective. A relative reduction in infarct volume in animal models is
the necessary and sufficient evidence required
to advance a drug into clinical trials. Repli-
cating these pre-clinical observations in a
clinical population is a logical step in clinical
drug development, but has often been ne-
glected. Treatments that do not lead to a
smaller infarct in patients relative to an untreated cohort are unlikely to show a clinical
benefit. Performing a dose escalation safety
study, followed by large clinical endpoint
trials at the maximum tolerated dose in the
absence of evidence that the drug has the target biological effect in patients that it had in
the animal models has been tried and failed
for treatments beyond the three hour time
window. Pilot proof-of-principle studies toward defining the optimal sample on a bio-
logically meaningful outcome variable are an
important step.

Ordinarily a drug must have a beneficial
effect on a clinical endpoint or on a validated
surrogate endpoint to demonstrate effectiveness and lead to registration. Current regulations governing the United States Food and
Drug Administration state that a drug that
has the potential to address unmet medical
needs for serious and life-threatening conditions, such as stroke, may be approved if it
has an effect on a surrogate endpoint that is
reasonably likely to predict clinical benefit.
Such surrogate endpoints are considered to be
not validated because, while suggestive of
clinical benefit, their relationship to clinical
outcomes is not proven. The internationally
accepted regulatory standards of the International Conference on Harmonization also
state that surrogate endpoints may be used as
primary endpoints when the surrogate is reasonably likely to predict clinical outcome.
Change in volume of ischemic brain injury

using DWI and T2-WI has been proposed as
a surrogate marker of clinical outcome in
stroke trials. Much of the thought on the use
of biomarkers as measures of drug activity
and potential surrogates have come from
fields, such as oncology or cardiology, where
death or a comparably objective and reliable
assessment is the relevant clinical endpoint.
For these disease categories, the biomarker
does not fully capture the pathology underlying of the disease as well as the clinical endpoint does. Principles of the use of biomarkers and potential surrogates are different for
brain disorders in which disability defined by
imperfect clinical rating scales rather than
death is the relevant clinical variable, and in
which the biomarker – macroscopic brain lesion – more fully captures the pathology than
the clinical scales. Stroke is a special case
among brain diseases because 1) it is a single
event that is not progressive beyond the initial hours and days, 2) there is a high rate of
spontaneous clinical recovery (implying that
clinical improvement is less reflective of drug
effect), 3) it requires rapid diagnosis under
emergency conditions (the diagnostic certainty is less), and 4) a single discrete lesion
fully captures the pathology (the clinical
manifestations result from the size and location of the ischemic damage). For stroke the
true clinical endpoint, disability, is difficult to
measure, and can only approximated by clinical scales. Furthermore, experts do not agree
on how to measure outcome using clinical
scales, and the criterion of 'complete recovery' used in many trials may include patients
with significant disability. For these reasons,
lesion volume as a biomarker is likely to be
more helpful for stroke than in cancer and
cardiac disorders.

MRI measurements of lesion volume
acutely and chronically have proven to be a
marker of clinical severity measured by stroke
scales [15, 26, 205, 352] and changes in lesion
volume over time are associated with change
in clinical severity [377]. The two citicoline
DWI stroke trials both measured DWI within
24 hours of onset and T2-WI at week 12. Volume measurements were performed in a central lab by a single reader blinded to clinical
information and treatment assignment. Both
protocols defined clinical improvement a

priori as an improvement on NIHSS of 7 or more points. Exploratory analyses in the first trial (010; n = 81) led to planned confirmatory analyses in the second trial (018; n = 133). In both trials, the association of volume change to clinical improvement was highly significant (P < 0.0001), and patients who improved had decreased volume change relative to those who did not (P < 0.01). The positive predictive value of a reduction in lesion volume predicting clinical improvement was 66% for the 010 trial and 76% for the 018 trial; the negative predictive values were 73% and 52%, respectively. The sensitivity of lesion volume decrease for detection of clinical improvement was 74% for the 010 trial and 70% for the 018 trial; the specificities were 64% and 60%, respectively. These results confirm that the change in lesion volume is a marker of clinical improvement in patients in these trials and probably a better marker than the respective DWI or PWI lesion volumes alone [302]. Results on this marker in these and other trials have been consistent with results on clinical measures. Based upon the results of these trials, the regulatory standard is met: there is sufficient evidence to recommend MRI volume change as a surrogate endpoint that is reasonably likely to predict clinical outcome in stroke trials. Although surrogates not yet validated may be used if reasonably likely to predict the outcome, eventual validation is a goal.

The factors required for validation of MRI as a surrogate marker are summarized in Table 14.3. The first four of these requirements have been met. Confirmation of the validity of many of these features of DWI and PWI in acute stroke has recently come from the first prospective multi-center stroke trial using MRI as an inclusion and primary outcome measure, the citicoline MRI stroke trial [377]. The fifth criterion of validation – the concordance of effects on clinical outcomes and surrogate outcomes, continues to be evaluated in ongoing trials. Effective drugs should show benefit on both clinical and imaging outcome measures. To date several stroke trials have used stroke MRI and the results seem concordant with respect to the clinical endpoints. Table 14.4 summarizes these results.

Table 14.3. Requirements of a validated surrogate for DWI and PWI

1. DWI and PWI as biologic markers of the disease process in ischemic stroke
2. The tests are sensitive and specific for the diagnosis of stroke in patients
3. Lesion volumes correlate with clinical function as measured by clinical rating scales, predict outcome, and co-vary over time with clinical severity and clinical changes
4. Rational co-variates affecting lesion volume outcomes identified
5. Utility in identifying effective treatments in trials proven

To fully establish diffusion and perfusion MRI as a validated surrogate in stroke trials several conditions need to be satisfied (the first four have been met, sufficient to meet the regulatory requirement for surrogate use of 'reasonably likely to predict outcome' on clinical variables)

Table 14.4. Concordance of MRI and clinical results in clinical trials

Trials	Clinical benefit	MR Surrogate benefit	MR Natural history
i.v. tPA (0–3 h)	+	(+)	+
i.v. tPA (3–6 h)	– (+ secondary EP)	(+)	+
i.a. t-lysis	+	–	+
Citicoline	– (+ secondary)	+	+
GAIN	–	–	–
POST	–	–	–

No randomized clinical trial with thrombolytic therapy using MRI has been reported, however for those therapies Table 14.4 lists results from natural history studies. The citicoline trials provide support for this wherein trends on clinical and effects on imaging outcomes measures have been observed [67–69, 377, 378]. Ineffective drugs will show benefit on neither clinical nor imaging outcome measures. The latter has been found for the GAIN and POST neuroprotective trials, which showed no effect on clinical or MRI surrogate outcomes [197, 292, 374, 375].

If the results on clinical endpoints and imaging endpoints were to be discordant, what are the possible explanations? If lesion volume shows a benefit but the clinical endpoint does not, the most likely explanation would be that the trial design or the choice of clinical endpoints is insensitive to the drug effect or that there is a toxicity affecting the measurement of clinical outcome that offsets the neuroprotective effect of the therapy. If clinical endpoint shows a benefit but lesion volume does not, this could either be that the imaging methods are insensitive to the drug effect or that the clinical benefit is not mediated by a direct effect on the evolving infarct. The latter possibility is not relevant to reperfusion or neuroprotective therapies, but may apply to classes of drugs that, for example, treat post-stroke mood disorders or would lead to enhanced recovery through functional reorganization. This comparison is only meaningful if studies are optimally designed and equally powered to show effect on their respective outcome measures, i.e., the optimal sample size for imaging studies may be too small to show clinical effects. Full validation must eventually be proven, but as we see from the regulatory standards it is not required in order to use lesion volume by MRI as a surrogate outcome in stroke trials. An imaging benefit may never stand alone as a surrogate, since there must also be evidence of clinical benefit. One could imagine a small but statistically significant volume reduction that would have a trivial or undetectable clinical effect. However, a benefit on the surrogate may be acceptable as an independent source of confirmatory data in support of benefit seen in clinical endpoint trials, but an application for registration of a stroke drug using MRI outcomes has not yet been submitted to regulatory agencies.

The pharmaceutical industry has taken the initiative investigating this final step in validation. The results of several industry-sponsored drug trials using MRI as a surrogate will be known over the next several years, and those studies should provide the most decisive information regarding the utility of MRI as a surrogate outcome measure in stroke trials. Several others are in progress (Table 14.5).

Table 14.5. Ongoing acute stroke trials using MRI (winter 2002)

Trial Acronym	Intervention	Time window
Thrombolysis studies		
EPITHET	i.v. tPA	3–6 h
DEFUSE	i.v. tPA	3–6 h
DIAS	i.v. desmoteplase	3–9 h
MR SELECT	i.a. tPA	6–12 h
ROSIE	i.v. abciximab/reteplase	3–24 h
Neuroprotection studies		
ARTIST MRI	i.v. AMPA antagonist	0–6 h
MR IMAGES	i.v. magnesium	0–12 h
SIS	i.v. sipatragine	0–12 h
COOL-AID I	hypothermia (i.v. catheter)	0–12 h

Table 14.6. Sample features of MRI-based stroke trials

MRI sequences
- DWI: parenchymal injury
- PWI: hemodynamic abnormality
- MRA: arterial occlusion
- GRE: hemorrhage detection
- FLAIR: chronic and subacute lesions

Selection criteria
- Cortical DWI lesion >5 ml
- PWI/DWI-mismatch
- No pre-existing lesions in same vascular territory

Outcome variables
- Lesion volume change pre to post treatment
  - Absolute change
  - Percentage change
  - Proportion of patients reaching change criterion (e.g., volume decrease)
- Final lesion volume on high resolution FLAIR at day 30 with baseline DWI volume of abnormality as a co-variate

Data analysis
- Approach to non-normal distribution of lesion volumes
  - Transformed lesion volume (percentage change, log, cube root)
  - Non-parametric statistical model
- Co-variance analysis on baseline variables
  - NIHSS
  - Volume of hypoperfusion
  - Initial lesion volume
  - Others?
    - Age
    - Time to treatment

There have been concerns raised in the past that the use of stroke MRI in stroke clinical trials is impractical for technical and logistical reasons (e.g., scan duration and availability). The practical limitations have disappeared with the widespread availability of ultrafast echoplanar imaging with diffusion and perfusion capability on commercial MRI scanners. A highly motivated, well-coordinated center can perform emergency diffusion and perfusion MRI with a latency to scan and scanning session duration approaching that of emergency head CT. There are now well over 100 centers worldwide that are capable and experienced in performing these types of acute MR exams in clinical trials. Key design issues with regard to the use of DWI and PWI in stroke trials are proposed in Table 14.6.

MRI-based recruitment into trials with time window of six hours have proven feasible, as has specifically selection based on lesion size, location, and the PWI/DWI-mismatch. As the field of stroke clinical trials examines opportunities for improving trial design, positive imaging diagnoses in patient selection and use of imaging as treatment assessments is assuming a more and more useful role. MRI is increasingly used as a selection tool and an outcome measure in stroke trials, reflecting recognition that direct pathophysiological imaging may provide a more rational approach to stroke therapy. Patient selection and outcomes based exclusively on clinical assessment and non-hemorrhagic CT scans may no longer be appropriate for all stroke trials.

References

1. Abe T, Kazama M, Naito I (1981) Clinical evaluation for efficacy of tissue cultured urokinase (TCUK) on cerebral thrombosis by means of multi-centre double blind study (Translated from Japanese). Blood-Vessel 12: 321–341

2. Albers GW (1999) Expanding the window for thrombolytic therapy in acute stroke – the potential role of acute MRI for patient selection. Stroke 30: 2230–2237

3. Albers GW, Bates VE, Clark WM, Bell R, Verro P, Hamilton SA (2000) Intravenous tissue-type plasminogen activator for treatment of acute stroke: the Standard Treatment with Alteplase to Reverse Stroke (STARS) study. Jama 283(9): 1145–1150

4. Alexander JA, Sheppard S, Davis PC, Salverda P (1996) Adult cerebrovascular diseases: role of modified rapid fluid attenuated inversion-recovery sequences. AJNR Am J Neuroradiol 17: 1507–1513

5. Alexandrov AV, Burgin WS, Demchuk AM, El-Mitwalli A, Grotta JC (2001) Speed of intracranial clot lysis with intravenous tissue plasminogen activator therapy: sonographic classification and short-term improvement. Circulation 103(24): 2897–2902

6. Alexandrov AV, Masdeu JC, Devous Sr MD, Black SE, Grotta JC (1997) Brain single-photon emission CT with HMPAO and safety of thrombolytic therapy in acute ischemic stroke. Proceedings of the meeting of the SPECT Safe Thrombolysis Study Collaborators and the members of the Brain Imaging Council of the Society of Nuclear Medicine. Stroke 28(9): 1830–1834

7. Arnold M, Schroth G, Nedeltchev K, Loher T, Remonda L, Stepper F, Sturzenegger M, Mattle HP (2002) Intra-arterial thrombolysis in 100 patients with acute stroke due to middle cerebral artery occlusion. Stroke 33(7): 1828–1833

8. Astrup J, Siesjö B, Symon L (1981) Thresholds in cerebral ischemia – the ischemic penumbra. Stroke 12: 723–725

9. Atarashi J, Ohtomo E, Araki G, Itoh E, Togi H, Matsuda T (1985) Clinical utility of urokinase in the treatment of acute stage cerebral thrombosis: multi-center double blind study in comparison with placebo (Translated from Japanese). Clin Eval 13: 659–709

10. Atlas SW (1993) MR imaging is highly sensitive for acute subarachnoid hemorrhage ... not! Radiology 186(2): 319–322; discussion 323

11. Atlas SW, Thulborn KR (1998) MR detection of hyperacute parenchymal hemorrhage of the brain. AJNR Am J Neuroradiol 19: 1471–1477

12. Auer LM, Deinsberger W, Niederkorn K, Gell G, Kleinert R, Schneider G, Holzer P, Bone G, Mokry M, Korner E, et al. (1989) Endoscopic surgery versus medical treatment for spontaneous intracerebral hematoma: a randomized study. J Neurosurg 70(4): 530–535

13. Axel L (1980) Cerebral blood flow determination by rapid-sequence computed tomography. Radiology 137: 679–686

14. Baird AE, Benfield A, Schlaug G, Siewert B, Lovblad KO, Edelman RR, Warach S (1997) Enlargement of human cerebral ischemic lesion volumes measured by diffusion-weighted magnetic resonance imaging. Ann Neurol 41(5): 581–589

15. Baird AE, Lovblad KO, Dashe JF, Connor A, Burzynski C, Schlaug G, Straroselskaya I, Edelman RR, Warach S (2000) Clinical correlations of diffusion and perfusion lesion volumes in acute ischemic stroke. Cerebrovasc Dis 10(6): 441–448

16. Baird AE, Warach S (1999) Magnetic resonance imaging of acute stroke. J Cereb Blood Flow Met 18(6): 583–609

17. Bammer R, Fazekas F (2002) Diffusion imaging in multiple sclerosis. Neuroimaging Clin N Am 12(1): 71–106

18. Barber PA, Darby DG, Desmond PM, Yang Q, Gerraty RP, Jolley D, Donnan GA, Tress BM, Davis SM (1998) Prediction of stroke outcome with echoplanar perfusion- and diffusion-weighted MRI. Neurology 51: 418–426

19. Barber PA, Davis SM, Darby DG, Desmond PM, Gerraty RP, Yang Q, Jolley D, Donnan GA, Tress BM (1999) Absent middle cerebral artery flow predicts the presence and evolution of the ischemic penumbra. Neurology 52: 1125–1132

20. Barber PA, Demchuk AM, Zhang J, Buchan AM (2000) Validity and reliability of a quantitative computed tomography score in predicting outcome of hyperacute stroke before thrombolytic therapy. ASPECTS Study Group. Alberta Stroke Programme Early CT Score. Lancet 355(9216): 1670–1674

21. Barber PA, Zhang J, Demchuk AM, Hill MD, Buchan AM (2001) Why are stroke patients excluded from TPA therapy?: An analysis of patient eligibility. Neurology 56(8): 1015–1020

22. Barnwell SL, Clark WM, Nguyen TT, O'Neill OR, Wynn ML, Coull BM (1994) Safety and efficacy of delayed intraarterial urokinase therapy with mechanical clot disruption for thromboembolic stroke. AJNR Am J Neuroradiol 15(10): 1817–1822

23. Baron JC, vonKummer R, delZoppo GJ (1995) Treatment of acute ischemic stroke. Challenging the concept of a rigid and universal time window. Stroke 26: 2219–2221

24. Basser PJ, Pierpaoli C (1996) Microstructural and physiological features of tissues elucidated by quantitative-diffusion-tensor MRI. J Magn Reson B 111: 209–219

25. Baumgartner RW, Ringelstein EB (1996) Cerebrovascular ultrasound diagnosis. Ther Umsch 53(7): 528–534

26. Beaulieu C, de Crespigny A, Tong DC, Moseley ME, Albers GW, Marks MP (1999) Longitudinal magnetic resonance imaging study of perfusion and diffusion in stroke: evolution of lesion volume and correlation with clinical outcome. Ann Neurol 46(4): 568–578

27. Becker KJ, Monsein LH, Ulatowski J, Mirski M, Williams M, Hanley DF (1996) Intraarterial thrombolysis in vertebrobasilar occlusion. AJNR Am J Neuroradiol 17(2): 255–262

28. Benfield Y, Prasad PV, Edelman RR, Warach S (1996) On the optimal b value for measurement of lesion volumes in acute human stroke by diffusion weighted imaging, ISMRM, Fourth Scientific Meeting, Book of abstracts, 1996

29. Benner T, Heiland S, Erb G, Forsting M, Sartor K (1997) Accuracy of gamma-variate fits to concentration-time curves from dynamic susceptibility-contrast enhanced MRI: influence of time resolution, maximal signal drop and signal-to-noise. Magn Reson Imaging 15: 307–317

30. Benner T, Reimer P, Erb G, Schuierer G, Heiland S, Fischer C, Geens V, Sartor K, Forsting M (1998) Cerebral MR perfusion imaging: first clinical application of a 1 molar gadolinium chelate in a double-blinded randomized dose finding study, ISMRM, Sixth Scientific Meeting, Book of Abstracts, 1998

31. Benveniste H, Hedlund LW, Johnson GA (1992) Mechanism of detection of acute cerebral ischemia in rats by diffusion-weighted magnetic resonance microscopy. Stroke 23: 746–754

32. Berrouschot J, Barthel H, Hesse S, Knapp WH, Schneider D, von Kummer R (2000) Reperfusion and metabolic recovery of brain tissue and clinical outcome after ischemic stroke and thrombolytic therapy. Stroke 31(7): 1545–1551

33. Berrouschot J, Barthel H, Hesse S, Koster J, Knapp WH, Schneider D (1998) Differentiation between transient ischemic attack and ischemic stroke within the first six hours after onset of symptoms by using 99mTc-ECD-SPECT. J Cereb Blood Flow Metab 18(8): 921–929

34. Blackmore CC, Francis CW, Bryant RG, Brenner B, Marder VJ (1990) Magnetic resonance imaging of blood and clots in vitro. Invest Radiol 25(12): 1316–1324

35. Bozzao L, Angeloni U, Bastianello S, Fantozzi LM, Pierallini A, Fieschi C (1991) Early angiographic and CT findings in patients with hemorrhagic infarction in the distribution of the middle cerebral artery. AJNR Am J Neuroradiol 12(6): 1115–1121

36. Bozzao L, Bastianello S, Fantozzi LM, Angeloni U, Argentino C, Fieschi C (1989) Correlation of angiographic and sequential CT findings in patients with evolving cerebral infarction. AJNR Am J Neuroradiol 10(6): 1215–1222

37. Bradley WG, Jr. (1993) MR appearance of hemorrhage in the brain. Radiology 189(1): 15–26

38. Brandt T, Knauth M, Wildermuth S, Winter R, von Kummer R, Sartor K, Hacke W (1999) CT angiography and Doppler sonography for emergency assessment in acute basilar artery ischemia. Stroke 30(3): 606–612

39. Brandt T, Steinke W, Thie A, Pessin MS, Caplan LR (2000) Posterior cerebral artery territory infarcts: clinical features, infarct topography, causes and outcome. Multicenter results and a review of the literature. Cerebrovasc Dis 10(3): 170–182

40. Brandt T, von Kummer R, Muller Kuppers M, Hacke W (1996) Thrombolytic therapy of acute basilar artery occlusion. Variables affecting recanalization and outcome. Stroke 27(5): 875–881

41. Brant-Zawadzki M, Atkinson D, Detrick M, Bradley W, Seidmore GSJ (1996) Fluid-attenuated inversion recovery (FLAIR) for assessment of cerebral infarction. Initial clinical experience in 50 patients. Stroke 27: 1187–1191

42. Broderick JP, Shuaib A (2002) The Interventional Management of Stroke (IMS) Study: Preliminary Results, International Stroke Conference, San Antonio, Tx, USA, February 7–9th, 2002

43. Brooks RA, Di Chiro G, Patronas N (1989) MR imaging of cerebral hematomas at different field strengths: theory and applications. J Comput Assist Tomogr 13(2): 194–206

44. Brott T, Adams HP, Jr., Olinger CP, Marler JR, Barsan WG, Biller J, Spilker J, Holleran R, Eberle R, Hertzberg V, et al. (1989) Measurements of acute cerebral infarction: a clinical examination scale. Stroke 20(7): 864870

45. Brott T, Adams HP, Olinger CP, Marler JR, Barsan WG, Biller J, Spilker J, Holleran R, Eberle R, Hertzberg V, Walker M (1989) Developing measurements of acute cerebral infarction: a clinical examination scale. Stroke 20: 864–870

46. Brott TG (2002) A combined metaanalysis of NINDS, ECASS I and II, ATLANTIS, International Stroke Conference, San Antonio, Tx, USA, February 7–9th, 2002

47. Bruckmann H, Ferbert A, del Zoppo GJ, Hacke W, Zeumer H (1986) Acute vertebral-basilar thrombosis. Angiologic-clinical comparison and therapeutic implications. Acta Radiol Suppl 369: 38–42

48. Brückmann H, Jansen O (1996) Ischämische Hirnerkrankungen. In: Sartor K (ed) Neuroradiologie, Thieme Verlag, Stuttgart, New York

49. Bruhn H, Frahm J, Gyngell ML, Merboldt KD, Hanicke W, Sauter R (1989) Cerebral metabolism in man after acute stroke: new observations using localized proton NMR spectroscopy. Magn Reson Med 9: 126–131

50. Bruning R, Penzkofer H, Schopf U, Becker C, Mayer T, Spuler A, Berchtenbreiter C, Steiger HJ, Reiser M (1998) Calculation of absolute cerebral blood volume and cerebral blood flow by means of electron-beam computed tomography (EBT) in acute ischemia. Radiologe 38(12): 1054–1059

51. Bullock R, Brock Utne J, van Dellen J, Blake G (1988) Intracerebral hemorrhage in a primate model: effect on regional cerebral blood flow. Surg Neurol 29(2): 101–107

52. Busch E, Beaulieu C, de Crespigny A, Moseley ME (1998) Diffusion MR imaging during acute subarachnoid hemorrhage in rats. Stroke 29: 2155–2161

53. Buxton RB (1993) The diffusion sensitivity of fast steady state free precession imaging. Magn Reson Med 29: 235–243

54. Calamante F, Gadian DG, Connelly A (2000) Delay and dispersion effects in dynamic susceptibility contrast MRI: simulations using singular value decomposition. Magn Reson Res 44: 466–473

55. Calamante F, Gadian DG, Connelly A (2002) Quantification of perfusion using bolus tracking magnetic resonance imaging in stroke: assumptions, limitations, and potential implications for clinical use. Stroke 33(4): 1146–1151

56. Chakeres DW, Bryan RN (1986) Acute subarachnoid hemorrhage: in vitro comparison of magnetic resonance and computed tomography. AJNR Am J Neuroradiol 7(2): 223–228

57. Chalela JA, Ezzeddine MA, Calabrese TM, Latour LL, Baird AE, Luby ML, Warach S (2002) Diffusion and perfusion changes two hours after intravenous rt-PA therapy: a preliminary report. Stroke 33(1): 356–357

58. Chenevert TL, Pipe JG (1991) Effect of bulk tissue motion on quantitative perfusion and diffusion magnetic resonance imaging. Magn Reson Med 19: 261–265

59. Chin HY, Taber KH, Hayman LA (1991) Temporal changes in red blood cell hydration: application to MRI of hemorrhage. Neuroradiol 33(Suppl): 79–81

60. Chinese Acute Stroke Trial Collaborative Group (1997) CAST: randomised placebo-controlled trial of early aspirin use in 20000 patients with acute ischaemic stroke. Lancet 349 (June 7): 1641–1649

61. Chiu D, Krieger D, Villar-Cordova C, Kasner SE, Morgenstern LB, Bratina PL, Yatsu FM, Grotta JC (1998) Intravenous tissue plasminogen activator for acute ischemic stroke – feasibility, safety and efficacy in the first year of clinical practice. Stroke 29: 18–22

62. Christou I, Alexandrov AV, Burgin WS, Wojner AW, Felberg RA, Malkoff M, Grotta JC (2000) Timing of recanalization after tissue plasminogen activator therapy determined by transcranial Doppler correlates with clinical recovery from ischemic stroke. Stroke 31(8): 1812–1816

63. Chrysikopoulos H, Papanikolaou N, Pappas J, Papandreou A, Roussakis A, Vassilouthis J, Andreou J (1996) Acute subarachnoid haemorrhage: detection with magnetic resonance imaging. Br J Radiol 69(823): 601–609

64. Clark RA, Watanabe AT, Bradley Jr. WG, Roberts JD (1990) Acute hematoma: effects of deoxygenation, hematocrit, and fibrin clot formation and retraction on T2 shortening. Radiol 175: 201–206

65. Clark RK, Lee EV, White RF, Jonak ZL, Feuerstein GZ, Barone FC (1994) Reperfusion following focal stroke hastens inflammation and resolution of ischemic injured tissue. Brain Res Bull 35: 387–392

66. Clark WM, Albers GW, Madden KP, Hamilton S (2000) The rtPA (alteplase) 0- to 6-hour acute stroke trial, part A (A0276g): results of a double-blind, placebo-controlled, multicenter study. Thrombolytic therapy in acute ischemic stroke study investigators. Stroke 31(4): 811–816

67. Clark WM, Warach SJ, Pettigrew LC, Gammans RE, Sabounjian LA (1997) A randomized dose-response trial of citicoline in acute ischemic stroke patients. Citicoline Stroke Study Group. Neurology 49(3): 671–678

68. Clark WM, Wechsler LR, Sabounjian LA, Schwiderski UE (2001) A phase III randomized efficacy trial of 2000 mg citicoline in acute ischemic stroke patients. Neurology 57(9): 1595–1602

69. Clark WM, Williams BJ, Selzer KA, Zweifler RM, Sabounjian LA, Gammans RE (1999) A randomized efficacy trial of citicoline in pa-

tients with acute ischemic stroke. Stroke 30(12): 2592–2597

70. Clark WM, Wissman S, Albers GW, Jhamandas JH, Madden KP, Hamilton S (1999) Recombinant tissue-type plasminogen activator (Alteplase) for ischemic stroke 3 to 5 hours after symptom onset. The ATLANTIS Study: a randomized controlled trial. Alteplase Thrombolysis for Acute Noninterventional Therapy in Ischemic Stroke. JAMA 282(21): 2019–2026

71. Condette-Auliac S, Bracard S, Anxionnat R, Schmitt E, Lacour JC, Braun M, Meloneto J, Cordebar A, Yin L, Picard L (2001) Vasospasm after subarachnoid hemorrhage: interest in diffusion-weighted MR imaging. Stroke 32(8): 1818–1824

72. Cornu C, Boutitie F, Candelise L, Boissel JP, Donnan GA, Hommel M, Jaillard A, Lees KR (2000) Streptokinase in acute ischemic stroke: an individual patient data meta-analysis: the thrombolysis in acute stroke pooling project. Stroke 31(7): 1555–1560

73. Cote R, Battista RN, Wolfson CM, Hachinski V (1988) Stroke assessment scales: guidelines for development, validation, and reliability assessment. Can J Neurol Sci 15(3): 261–265

74. Crain MR, Yuh WTC, Greene GM, Loes DJ, Ryals TJ, Sato Y, Hart MN (1991) Cerebral ischemia: evaluation with contrast-enhanced MR imaging. AJNR Am J Neuroradiol 12: 631–639

75. Davis D, Ulatowski J, Eleff S, Izuta M, Mori S, Shungu D, van Zijl PC (1994) Rapid monitoring of changes in water diffusion coefficients during reversible ischemia in cat and rat brain. Magn Reson Med 31: 454–460

76. Davis SM, Donnan GA, Gerraty RP, Mitchell PJ, Fitt G, Bladin CF, Mc Neil JJ, Rosen D, Stewart-Wynne EG, Hankey GJ (1996) Australian Urokinase Stroke Trial (Abstract). Cerebrovasc Dis 6: 188

77. de Crespigny AJ, Marks MP, Enzmann DR, Moseley ME (1995) Navigated diffusion imaging of normal and ischemic human brain. Magn Reson Med 33: 720–728

78. Deinsberger W, Vogel J, Fuchs C, Auer LM, Kuschinsky W, Boker DK (1999) Fibrinolysis and aspiration of experimental intracerebral hematoma reduces the volume of ischemic brain in rats. Neurol Res 21(5): 517–523

79. del Zoppo GJ, Ferbert A, Otis S, Bruckmann H, Hacke W, Zyroff J, Harker LA, Zeumer H (1988) Local intra-arterial fibrinolytic therapy in acute carotid territory stroke. A pilot study. Stroke 19(3): 307–313

80. del Zoppo GJ, Higashida RT, Furlan AJ, Pessin MS, Rowley HA, Gent M, et al (1998) PROACT: a phase II randomized trial of recombinant pro-urokinase by direct arterial delivery in acute middle cerebral artery stroke. Stroke 29: 4–11

81. Dethy S, Goldman S, Blecic S, Luxen A, Levivier M, Hildebrand J (1994) Carbon-11-methionine and fluorine-18-FDG PET study in brain hematoma. J Nucl Med 35(7): 1162–1166

82. Doerfler A, Engelhorn T, von Kummer R, Weber J, Knauth M, Heiland S, Sartor K, Forsting M (1998) Are iodinated contrast agents detrimental in acute cerebral ischemia? An experimental study in rats. Radiology 206(1): 211–217

83. Donnan GA, Davis SM, Chambers BR, Gates PC, Hankey GJ, McNeil JJ, Rosen D, Stewart-Wynne EG, Tuck RR (1996) Streptokinase for acute ischemic stroke with relationship to time of administration: Australian Streptokinase (ASK) Trial Study Group. JAMA 276(12): 961–966

84. Ebisu T, Tanaka C, Umeda M, Kitamura M, Fukunaga M, Aoki I, Sato H, Higuchi T, Naruse S, Horikawa Y, Ueda S (1997) Hemorrhagic and nonhemorrhagic stroke: diagnosis with diffusion-weighted and T2-weighted echo-planar MR imaging. Radiology 203(3): 823–828

85. Evans AJ, Richardson DB, Tien R, Mac Fall JR, Hedlund LW, Heinz ER, Boyko O, Sostman HD (1993) Poststenotic signal loss in MR angiography: effects of echo time, flow compensation, and fractional echo. AJNR Am J Neuroradiol 14: 721–729

86. Ezura M, Kagawa S (1992) Selective and superselective infusion of urokinase for embolic stroke. Surg Neurol 38(5): 353–358

87. Fagan SC, Morgenstern LB, Petitta A, Ward RE, Tilley BC, Marler JR, Levine SR, Broderick JP, Kwiatkowski TG, Frankel M, Brott TG, Walker MD (1998) Cost-effectiveness of tissue plasminogen activator for acute ischemic stroke. NINDS rt-PA Stroke Study Group. Neurology 50(4): 883–890

88. Fazekas F, Kleinert R, Roob G, Kleinert G, Kapeller P, Schmidt R, Hartung HP (1999) Histopathologic analysis of foci of signal loss on gradient-echo T2*-weighted MR images in patients with spontaneous intracerebral hemorrhage: evidence of microangiopathy-related microbleeds. AJNR Am J Neuroradiol 20(4): 637–642

89. Felber S, Auer A, Wolf C, Schocke M, Golaszewski S, Amort B, zurNedden D (1999) MRI characteristics of spontaneous intracerebral hemorrhage. Radiologe 39(10): 838–846

90. Fernandes HM, Gregson B, Siddique S, Mendelow AD (2000) Surgery in intracerebral hemorrhage: the uncertainty continues. Stroke 31(10): 2511–2516

91. Fiebach JB, Jansen O, Schellinger PD, Heiland S, Hacke W, Sartor K (2002) Serial analysis of the apparent diffusion coefficient time course in human stroke. Neuroradiology 44: 294–298

92. Fiebach JB, Jansen O, Schellinger PD, Knauth M, Hartmann M, Heiland S, Ryssel H, Pohlers O, Hacke W, Sartor K (2001) Comparison of CT with diffusion-weighted MRI in patients with hyperacute stroke. Neuroradiology 43: 628–632

93. Fiebach JB, Schellinger PD, Geletneky K, Wilde P, Meyer M, Hacke W, Sartor K (2002) Stroke MRI in hyperacute subarachnoid hemorrhage in humans. AJNR Am J Neuroradiol (submitted for publication)

94. Fiebach JB, Schellinger PD, Jansen O, Meyer M, Wilde P, Bender J, Schramm P, Jüttler E, Öhler J, Hartmann M, Hähnel S, Knauth M, Hacke W, Sartor K (2002) CT and diffusion-weighted MR-imaging in randomized order: DWI results in higher accuracy and lower interrater variability in the diagnosis of hyperacute ischemic stroke. Stroke 33(9): 2206–2210

95. Fiehler J, Knab R, Reichenbach JR, Fitzek C, Weiller C, Rother J (2001) Apparent diffusion coefficient decreases and magnetic resonance imaging perfusion parameters are associated in ischemic tissue of acute stroke patients. J Cereb Blood Flow Metab 21(5): 577–584

96. Fink JN, Kumar S, Horkan C, Linfante I, Selim MH, Caplan LR, Schlaug G (2002) The stroke patient who woke up: clinical and radiological features, including diffusion and perfusion MRI. Stroke 33(4): 988–993

97. Fisel CR, Ackerman JL, Buxton RB, Garrido L, Belliveau JW, Rosen BR, Brady TJ (1991) MR contrast due to microscopically heterogeneous magnetic susceptibility: numerical simulations and applications to cerebral physiology. Magn Reson Med 17: 336–347

98. Fisher M, Albers GW (1999) Applications of diffusion-perfusion magnetic resonance imaging in acute ischemic stroke. Neurology 52: 1750–1756

99. Fleiss J (1981) Statistical Methods for Rates and Proportions. Wiley, New York, pp 211–236

100. Fox T, Hamann GF, Strittmatter M, Haass A, Hermes M, Piepgras U (1996) Local intraarterial fibrinolysis in vertebrobasilar thrombosis – prognostic criteria (Abstract). Cerebrovasc Dis 6: 186

101. Fujita N, Hirabuki N, Fujii K, Hashimoto T, Miura T, Sato T, Kozuka T (1994) MR imaging of middle cerebral artery stenosis and occlusion: value of MR angiography. AJNR Am J Neuroradiol 15: 335–341

102. Furlan A, Higashida R, Wechsler L, Gent M, Rowley H, Kase C, Pessin M, Ahuja A, Callahan F, Clark WM, Silver F, Rivera F (1999) Intra-arterial prourokinase for acute ischemic stroke. The PROACT II study: a randomized controlled trial. Prolyse in acute cerebral thromboembolism. JAMA 282(21): 2003–2011

103. Gass A, Röther J, Gaa J (1999) Diffusion- and perfusion-weighted MRI in cerebral ischaemia – Part 2: clinical applications. Akt Neurol 26(7): 309–317

104. Gerriets T, Postert T, Goertler M, Stolz E, Schlachetzki F, Sliwka U, Seidel G, Weber S, Kaps M (2000) DIAS I: duplex-sonographic assessment of the cerebrovascular status in acute stroke: a useful tool for future stroke trials. Stroke 31(10): 2342–2345

105. Gillard JH, Barker PB, van Zijl PC, Bryan RN, Oppenheimer SM (1996) Proton MR spectroscopy in acute middle cerebral artery stroke. AJNR Am J Neuroradiol 17(5): 873–886

106. Gilman S (1998) Imaging the brain. First of two parts. N Engl J Med 338(12): 812–820

107. Gilman S (1998) Imaging the brain. Second of two parts. N Engl J Med 338(13): 889–896

108. Ginsberg MD, Pulsinelli WA (1994) The ischemic penumbra, injury thresholds, and the therapeutic window for acute stroke. Ann Neurol 36(4): 553–554

109. Gomori JM, Grossman RI (1988) Mechanisms responsible for the MR appearance and evolution of intracranial hemorrhage. Radiographics 8(3): 427–440

110. Gomori JM, Grossman RI, Goldberg HI, Zimmerman RA, Bilaniuk LT (1985) Intracranial hematomas: imaging by high-field MR. Radiology 157(1): 87–93

111. Gomori JM, Grossman RI, Yu-Ip C, Asakura T (1987) NMR relaxation times of blood: dependence on field strength, oxidation state, and cell integrity. J Comput Assist Tomogr 11(4): 684–690

112. Gonner F, Remonda L, Mattle H, Sturzenegger M, Ozdoba C, Lovblad KO, Baumgartner R, Bassetti C, Schroth G (1998) Local intra-arterial thrombolysis in acute ischemic stroke. Stroke 29(9): 1894–1900

113. Gonzales RG, Schaefer PW, Buonanno FS, Schwamm LH, Budzik RF, Rordorf G, Wang B, Sorensen AG, Koroshetz WJ (1999) Diffusion-weighted MR imaging: diagnostic accuracy in patients imaged within 6 hours of stroke symptom onset. Radiology 210(1): 155–162

114. Grandin CB, Duprez TP, Smith AM, Mataigne F, Peeters A, Oppenheim C, Cosnard G (2001) Usefulness of magnetic resonance-derived quantitative measurements of cerebral blood flow and volume in prediction of infarct growth in hyperacute stroke. Stroke 32(5): 1147–1153

115. Granger CV, Cotter AC, Hamilton BB, Fiedler RC (1993) Functional assessment scales: a study of persons after stroke. Arch Phys Med Rehabil 74(2): 133–138

116. Griffiths PD, Wilkinson ID, Mitchell P, Patel MC, Paley MN, Romanowski CA, Powell TJ,

Hodgson TJ, Hoggard N, Jellinek D (2001) Multimodality MR imaging depiction of hemodynamic changes and cerebral ischemia in subarachnoid hemorrhage. AJNR Am J Neuroradiol 22(9): 1690–1697

117. Grond M, Rudolf J, Schmulling S, Stenzel C, Neveling M, Heiss WD (1998) Early intravenous thrombolysis with recombinant tissue-type plasminogen activator in vertebrobasilar ischemic stroke. Arch Neurol 55(4): 466–469

118. Grond M, Stenzel C, Schmulling S, Rudolf J, Neveling M, Lechleuthner A, Schneweis S, Heiss WD (1998) Early intravenous thrombolysis for acute ischemic stroke in a community-based approach. Stroke 29(8): 1544–1549

119. Grossman RI, Gomori JM, Goldberg HI, Hackney DB, Atlas SW, Kemp SS, Zimmerman RA, Bilaniuk LT (1988) MR imaging of hemorrhagic conditions of the head and neck. Radiographics 8(3): 441–454

120. Grossman RI, Kemp SS, Ip CY, Fishman JE, Gomori JM, Joseph PM, Asakura T (1986) Importance of oxygenation in the appearance of acute subarachnoid hemorrhage on high field magnetic resonance imaging. Acta Radiol Suppl 369(1): 56–58

121. Grotta J (1997) Should thrombolytic therapy be the first-line treatment for acute ischemic stroke? N Engl J Med 337: 1309–1310

122. Gruber A, Nasel C, Lang W, Kitzmuller E, Bavinzski G, Czech T (2000) Intra-arterial thrombolysis for the treatment of perioperative childhood cardioembolic stroke. Neurology 54(8): 1684–1686

123. Gustafsson O, Rossitti S, Ericsson A, Raininko R (1999) MR imaging of experimentally induced intracranial hemorrhage in rabbits during the first 6 hours. Acta Radiol 40(4): 360–368

124. Hacke W, Brott T, Caplan L, Meier D, Fieschi C, von Kummer R, Donnan G, Heiss WD, Wahlgren NG, Spranger M, Boysen G, Marler JR (1999) Thrombolysis in acute ischemic stroke: controlled trials and clinical experience. Neurology 53(7): S3–14

125. Hacke W, Kaste M, Fieschi C, Toni D, Lesaffre E, von Kummer R, Boysen G, Bluhmki E, Hoexter G, Mahagne MH, Hennerici M (1995) Intravenous thrombolysis with recombinant tissue plasminogen activator for acute hemispheric stroke. The European Cooperative Acute Stroke Study. JAMA 274: 1017–1025

126. Hacke W, Kaste M, Fieschi C, von Kummer R, Davalos A, Meier D, Larrue V, Bluhmki E, Davis S, Donnan G, Schneider D, Diez-Tejedor E, Trouillas P (1998) Randomised double-blind placebo-controlled trial of thrombolytic therapy with intravenous alteplase in acute isch-

aemic stroke (ECASS II). Lancet 352: 1245–1251

127. Hacke W, Schwab S, DeGeorgia M (1994) Intensive care of acute ischemic stroke. Cerebrovasc Dis 4: 384–392

128. Hacke W, Schwab S, Horn M, Spranger M, De Georgia M, von Kummer R (1996) 'Malignant' middle cerebral artery territory infarction: clinical course and prognostic signs. Arch Neurol 53(4): 309–315

129. Hacke W, Steiner T, Schwab S (1996) Critical management of the acute stroke: medical and surgical therapy. In: Batjer HH, Caplan LR, Freiberg L, Greenlee RG Jr, Kopitnik TH Jr, Young WL (eds) Cerebrovascular disease, 1. ed, Lippincott-Raven, Hagerstown, pp 523–533

130. Hacke W, Stingele R, Steiner T, Schuchardt V, Schwab S (1995) Critical care of acute ischemic stroke. Intensive Care Med 21(10): 856–862

131. Hacke W, Warach S (2000) Diffusion-weighted MRI as an evolving standard of care in acute stroke. Neurology 54(8): 1548–1549

132. Hacke W, Willig V, Steiner T (1997) Update on thrombolytic therapy in ischemic stroke. Fibrinolysis & Proteolysis 11(Suppl. 2): 1–4

133. Hacke W, Zeumer H, Ferbert A, Brückmann H, DelZoppo G (1988) Intraarterial thrombolytic therapy improves outcome in patients with acute vertebrobasilar occlusive disease. Stroke 19: 1216–1222

134. Hadeishi H, Suzuki A, Yasui N, Hatazawa J, Shimosegawa E (2002) Diffusion-weighted magnetic resonance imaging in patients with subarachnoid hemorrhage. Neurosurgery 50(4): 741–747

135. Hagen T (1999) Intracerebral hemorrhage in the context of amyloid angiopathy. Radiologe 39(10): 847–854

136. Hajnal JV, Bryant DJ, Kasuboski L, Pattany PM, De Coene B, Lewis PD, Pennock JM, Oatridge A, Young IR, GM GMB (1992) Use of fluid attenuated inversion recovery (FLAIR) pulse sequences in MRI of the brain. J Comput Assist Tomogr 16: 841–844

137. Haley EC, Jr., Brott TG, Sheppard GL, Barsan W, Broderick J, Marler JR, Kongable GL, Spilker J, Massey S, Hansen CA, et al. (1993) Pilot randomized trial of tissue plasminogen activator in acute ischemic stroke. The TPA Bridging Study Group. Stroke 24(7): 1000–1004

138. Hamberg LM, Hunter GJ, Halpern EF, Hoop B, Gazelle GS, Wolf GL (1996) Quantitative high-resolution measurement of cerebrovascular physiology with slip-ring CT. AJNR Am J Neuroradiol 17(4): 639–650

139. Hamberg LM, Hunter GJ, Kierstead D, Lo EH, Gilberto-Gonzalez R, Wolf GL (1996) Measurement of cerebral blood volume with subtrac-

tion three-dimensional functional CT. AJNR Am J Neuroradiol 17(10): 1861–1869

140. Hamberg LM, Macfarlane R, Tasdemiroglu E, Boccalini P, Hunter GJ, Belliveau JW, Moskowitz MA, Rosen BR (1994) Measurement of cerebrovascular changes in cats after transient ischemia using dynamic magnetic resonance imaging. Stroke 24: 444–450

141. Handschu R, Garling A, Heuschmann PU, Kolominsky-Rabas PL, Erbguth F, Neundorfer B (2001) Acute stroke management in the local general hospital. Stroke 32: 866–870

142. Hartmann M, Heiland S, Sartor K (2002) [Functional MRI procedures in the diagnosis of brain tumors: Perfusion- and diffusion-weighted imaging]. Rofo Fortschr Geb Rontgenstr Neuen Bildgeb Verfahr 174(8): 955–964

143. Hayman LA, Pagani JJ, Kirkpatrick JB, Hinck VC (1989) Pathophysiology of acute intracerebral and subarachnoid hemorrhage: applications to MR imaging. AJR Am J Roentgenol 153(1): 135–139

144. Hayman LA, Taber KH, Ford JJ, Bryan RN (1991) Mechanisms of MR signal alteration by acute intracerebral blood: old concepts and new theories. AJNR Am J Neuroradiol 12(5): 899–907

145. Heiland S, Benner T, Reith W, Forsting M, Sartor K (1997) Perfusion-weighted MRI using gadobutrol as a contrast agent in a rat stroke model. J Magn Reson Imaging 7(6): 1109–1115

146. Heiland S, Reith W, Forsting M, Sartor K (1997) Diffusionsgewichtete MR-Tomographie bei fokaler zerebraler Ischämie: Möglichkeiten an einem 1.0 T Klinikgerät. Rofo Fortschr Geb Rontgenstr Neuen Bildgeb Verfahr 167: 297–303

147. Heiss WD, Grond M, Thiel A, von Stockhausen HM, Rudolf J, Ghaemi M, Lottgen J, Stenzel C, Pawlik G (1998) Tissue at risk of infarction rescued by early reperfusion: a positron emission tomography study in systemic recombinant tissue plasminogen activator thrombolysis of acute stroke. J Cereb Blood Flow Met 18(12): 1298–1307

148. Higashida RT, Halbach VV, Barnwell SL, Dowd CF, Hieshima GB (1994) Thrombolytic therapy in acute stroke. J Endovasc Surg 1: 4–15

149. Higashida RT, Halbach VV, Tsai FY, Dowd CF, Hieshima GB (1994) Interventional neurovascular techniques for cerebral revascularization in the treatment of stroke. Am J Roentgenol 163(4): 793–800

150. Higer HP, Pedrosa P, Schaeben W, Bielke G, Meindl S (1989) Intracranial hemorrhage in MRT. Radiologe 29(6): 297–302

151. Higuchi T, Fernandez EJ, Maudsley AA, Shimizu H, Weiner MW, Weinstein PR (1996) Mapping of lactate and N-acetyl-L-aspartate pre-

dicts infarction during acute focal ischemia: in vivo 1H magnetic resonance spectroscopy in rats. Neurosurgery 38(1): 121–129

152. Hirano T, Read SJ, Abbott DF, Sachinidis JI, Tochon-Danguy HJ, Egan GF, Bladin CF, Scott AM, McKay WJ, Donnan GA (1999) No evidence of hypoxic tissue on 18F-fluoromisonidazole PET after intracerebral hemorrhage. Neurology 53: 2179–2182

153. Hoehn-Berlage M, Eis M, Back T, Kohno K, Yamashita K (1995) Changes of relaxation times (T1, T2) and apparent diffusion coefficient after permanent middle cerebral artery occlusion in the rat: temporal evolution, regional extent, and comparison with histology. Magn Reson Med 34: 824–834

154. Horowitz SH, Zito JL, Donnarumma R, Patel M, Alvir J (1991) Computed tomographic-angiographic findings within the first five hours of cerebral infarction. Stroke 22(10): 1245–1253

155. International Stroke Trial Collaborative Group (1997) The International Stroke Trial (IST): a randomised trial of aspirin, subcutaneous heparin, both or neither among 19435 patients with acute ischaemic stroke. Lancet 349: 1569–1581

156. Jäger HR, Mansmann U, Hausmann O, Partzsch U, Moseley IF, Taylor WJ (2000) MRA versus digital subtraction angiography in acute subarachnoid haemorrhage: a blinded multireader study of prospectively recruited patients. Neuroradiology 42(5): 313–326

157. Janick PA, Hackney DB, Grossman RI, Asakura T (1991) MR imaging of various oxidation states of intracellular and extracellular hemoglobin. AJNR Am J Neuroradiol 12(5): 891–897

158. Jansen O, Heiland S, Schellinger P (1998) Neuroradiological diagnosis in acute ischemic stroke. Value of modern techniques. Nervenarzt 69: 465–471

159. Jansen O, Knauth M, Sartor K (1999) Advances in clinical neuroradiology. Akt Neurologie 26: 1–7

160. Jansen O, Schellinger PD, Fiebach JB, Hacke W, Sartor K (1999) Early recanalization in acute ischemic stroke saves tissue at risk defined by MRI. Lancet 353: 2036–2037

161. Jansen O, von Kummer R, Forsting M, Hacke W, Sartor K (1995) Thrombolytic therapy in acute occlusion of the intracranial internal carotid artery bifurcation. AJNR Am J Neuroradiol 16(10): 1977–1986

162. Jenkins A, Hadley DM, Teasdale GM, Condon B, Macpherson P, Patterson J (1988) Magnetic resonance imaging of acute subarachnoid hemorrhage. J Neurosurg 68(5): 731–736

163. Jennett B, Bond M (1975) Assessment of outcome after severe brain damage. Lancet 1(7905): 480–484

164. Johnson BA, Heisermann JE, Drayer BP, Keller PJ (1994) Intracranial MR angiography: its role in the integrated approach to brain infarction. AJNR Am J Neuroradiol 15: 901–908

165. Johnson KM, Tao JZT, Kennan RP, Gore JC (2000) Intravascular susceptibility agent effects on tissue transverse relaxation rates in vivo. Magn Reson Med 44: 909–914

166. Jorgensen HS, Nakayama H, Raaschou HO, Olsen TS (1995) Intracerebral hemorrhage versus infarction: stroke severity, risk factors, and prognosis. Ann Neurol 38: 45–50

167. Junghans U, Seitz RJ, Wittsack HJ, Aulich A, Siebler M (2001) Treatment of acute basilar artery thrombosis with a combination of systemic alteplase and tirofiban, a nonpeptide platelet glycoprotein IIb/IIIa inhibitor: report of four cases. Radiology 221(3): 795–801

168. Jungreis CA, Wechsler LR, Horton JA (1989) Intracranial thrombolysis via a catheter embedded in the clot. Stroke 20(11): 1578–1580

169. Kanno T, Nagata J, Nonomura K, Asai T, Inoue T, Nakagawa T, Mitsuyama F (1993) New approaches in the treatment of hypertensive intracerebral hemorrhage. Stroke 24(12 Suppl): I96–100

170. Katzan IL, Furlan AJ, Lloyd LE, Frank JI, Harper DL, Hinchey JA, Hammel JP, Qu A, Sila CA (2000) Use of tissue-type plasminogen activator for acute ischemic stroke: the Cleveland area experience. Jama 283(9): 1151–1158

171. Kidwell CS, Alger JR, F Di Salle, Starkman S, Villablanca P, Bentson J, Saver JL (1999) Diffusion MRI in patients with transient ischemic attacks. Stroke 30: 1174–1180

172. Kidwell CS, Saver JL, Carneado J, Sayre J, Starkman S, Duckwiler G, Gobin YP, Jahan R, Vespa P, Villablanca JP, Liebeskind DS, Vinuela F (2002) Predictors of hemorrhagic transformation in patients receiving intra-arterial thrombolysis. Stroke 33(3): 717–724

173. Kidwell CS, Saver JL, Mattiello J, Starkman S, Vinuela F, Duckwiler G, Gobin YP, Jahan R, Vespa P, Kalafut M, Alger JR (2000) Thrombolytic reversal of acute human cerebral ischemic injury shown by diffusion/perfusion magnetic resonance imaging. Ann Neurol 47(4): 462–469

174. Kidwell CS, Saver JL, Mattiello J, Warach S, Liebeskind DS, Starkman S, Vespa PM, Villablanca JP, Martin NA, Frazee J, Alger JR (2001) Diffusion-perfusion MR evaluation of perihematomal injury in hyperacute intracerebral hemorrhage. Neurology 57(9): 1611–1617

175. Kidwell CS, Saver JL, Villablanca JP, Duckwiler G, Fredieu A, Gough K, Leary MC, Starkman S, Gobin YP, Jahan R, Vespa P, Liebeskind DS,

176. Alger JR, Vinuela F (2002) Magnetic resonance imaging detection of microbleeds before thrombolysis: an emerging application. Stroke 33(1): 95–98

176. Kirkpatrick JB, Hayman LA (1992) Pathophysiology of intracranial hemorrhage. Neuroimaging Clin N Amer 2: 11–23

177. Knauth M, Forsting M, Hartmann M, Heiland S, Balzer T, Sartor K (1996) MR enhancement of brain lesions: increased contrast dose compared with magnetization transfer. Am J Neuroradiol 17(10): 1853–1859

178. Knauth M, Kummer Rv, Jansen O, Haehnel S, Doerfler A, Sartor K (1997) Potential of CT angiography in acute ischemic stroke. AJNR Am J Neuroradiol 18: 1001–1010

179. Knight RA, Dereski MO, Helpern JA, Ordidge RJ, Chopp M (1994) Magnetic resonance imaging assessment of evolving focal cerebral ischemia. Comparison with histopathology in rats. Stroke 25: 1252–1261

180. Koenig M, Banach-Planchamp R, Kraus M, Klotz E, Falk A, Gehlen W, Heuser L (2000) CT perfusion imaging in acute ischemic cerebral infarct: comparison of cerebral perfusion maps and conventional CT findings. Röfo Fortschr Geb Röntgenstr Neuen Bildgeb Verfahr 172: 219–226

181. Koenig M, Klotz E, Luka B, Venderink DJ, Spittler JF, Heuser L (1998) Perfusion CT of the brain: diagnostic approach for early detection of ischemic stroke. Radiology 209(1): 85–93

182. Koenig M, Kraus M, Theek C, Klotz E, Gehlen W, Heuser L (2001) Quantitative assessment of the ischemic brain by means of perfusion-related parameters derived from perfusion CT. Stroke 32(2): 431–437

183. Korogi Y, Takahashi M, Nakagawa T, Mabuchi N, Watabe T, Shiokawa Y, Shiga H, O'Uchi T, Miki H, Horikawa Y, Fujiwara S, Furuse M (1997) Intracranial vascular stenosis and occlusion: MR angiographic findings. Am J Neuroradiol 18: 135–143

184. Koroshetz WJ, Gonzalez G (1997) Diffusion-weighted MRI: an ECG for "brain attack"? Ann Neurol 41(5): 565–566

185. Kucharczyk J, Mintorovitch J, Asgari HS, Moseley ME (1991) Diffusion/perfusion imaging of acute cerebral ischemia. Magn Reson Med 19: 311–315

186. Kuker W, Thiex R, Rohde I, Rohde V, Thron A (2000) Experimental acute intracerebral hemorrhage. Value of MR sequences for a safe diagnosis at 1.5 and 0.5 T. Acta Radiol 41(6): 544–552

187. Kuschinsky W (1994) Blut-Hirn-Schranke, Liquor cerebrospinalis, Hirndurchblutung und Hirnstoffwechsel. In: Klinke R, Silbernagl S (eds) Lehrbuch der Physiologie, Thieme, Stuttgart, New York, pp 739–748

188. Kwiatkowski TG, Libman RB, Frankel M, Tilley BC, Morgenstern LB, Lu M, Broderick JP, Lewandowski CA, Marler JR, Levine SR, Brott T (1999) Effects of tissue plasminogen activator for acute ischemic stroke at one year. National Institute of Neurological Disorders and Stroke Recombinant Tissue Plasminogen Activator Stroke Study Group. N Engl J Med 340(23): 1781–1787

189. Kwong KK, McKinstry RC, Chien D, Crawley AP, Pearlman JD, Rosen BR (1991) CSF-suppressed quantitative single-shot diffusion imaging. Magn Reson Med 21: 157–163

190. Landis J, Koch G (1977) The measurement of observer agreement for categorial data. Biometrics 86: 974–977

191. Lansberg MG, Albers GW, Beaulieu C, Marks MP (2000) Comparison of diffusion-weighted MRI and CT in acute stroke. Neurology 54(8): 1557–1561

192. Latour LL, Svoboda K, Mitra PP, Sotak CH (1994) Time-dependent diffusion of water in a biological model system. Proc Natl Acad Sci U S A 91: 1229–1233

193. Laubach HJ, Jakob PM, Loevblad KO, Baird AE, Bovo MP, Edelman RR, Warach S (1998) A phantom for diffusion-weighted imaging of acute stroke. J Magn Reson Imaging 8(6): 1349–1354

194. Le Bihan D, Breton E, Lallemand D, Aubin ML, Vignaud J, Laval-Jeantet M (1988) Separation of diffusion and perfusion in intravoxel incoherent motion MR imaging. Radiology 168: 497–505

195. Le Bihan D, Breton E, Lallemand D, Grenier P, Cabanis E, Laval Jeantet M (1986) MR imaging of intravoxel incoherent motions: application to diffusion and perfusion in neurologic disorders. Radiology 161(2): 401–407

196. Le Bihan D, Turner R, Douek P, Patronas N (1992) Diffusion MR imaging: clinical applications. AJR Am J Roentgenol 159: 591–599

197. Lees KR, Asplund K, Carolei A, Davis SM, Diener HC, Kaste M, Orgogozo JM, Whitehead J (2000) Glycine antagonist (gavestinel) in neuroprotection (GAIN International) in patients with acute stroke: a randomised controlled trial. GAIN International Investigators. Lancet 355(9219): 1949–1954

198. Lev MH, Farkas J, Gemmete JJ, Hossain ST, Hunter GJ, Koroshetz WJ, Gonzalez RG (1999) Acute stroke: improved nonenhanced CT detection – benefits of soft-copy interpretation by using variable window width and center level settings. Radiology 213(1): 150–155

199. Lev MH, Nichols SJ (2000) Computed tomographic angiography and computed tomographic perfusion imaging of hyperacute stroke. Top Magn Reson Imaging 11: 273–287

200. Lev MH, Segal AZ, Farkas J, Hossain ST, Putman C, Hunter GJ, Budzik R, Harris GJ, Buonanno FS, Ezzeddine MA, Chang Y, Koroshetz WJ, Gonzalez RG, Schwamm LH (2001) Utility of perfusion-weighted CT imaging in acute middle cerebral artery stroke treated with intra-arterial thrombolysis: prediction of final infarct volume and clinical outcome. Stroke 32(9): 2021–2028

201. Lewandowski CA, Frankel M, Tomsick TA, Broderick J, Frey J, Clark W, Starkman S, Grotta J, Spilker J, Khoury J, Brott T (1999) Combined intravenous and intra-arterial r-TPA versus intra-arterial therapy of acute ischemic stroke: Emergency Management of Stroke (EMS) Bridging Trial. Stroke 30(12): 2598–2605

202. Leys D, Pruvo JP, Godefroy O, Rondepierre P, Leclerc X (1992) Prevalence and significance of hyperdense middle cerebral artery in acute stroke. Stroke 23(3): 317–324

203. Li F, Liu KF, Silva MD, Omae T, Sotak CH, Fenstermacher JD, Fisher M (2000) Transient and permanent resolution of ischemic lesions on diffusion-weighted imaging after brief periods of focal ischemia in rats: correlation with histopathology. Stroke 31(4): 946–954

204. Linfante I, Llinas RH, Caplan LR, Warach S (1999) MRI features of intracerebral hemorrhage within 2 hours from symptom onset. Stroke 30(11): 2263–2267

205. Lovblad KO, Baird AE, Schlaug G, Benfield A, Siewert B, Voetsch B, Connor A, Burzynski C, Edelman RR, Warach S (1997) Ischemic lesion volumes in acute stroke by diffusion-weighted magnetic resonance imaging correlate with clinical outcome. Ann Neurol 42(2): 164–170

206. Lubezky N, Fajer S, Barmeir E, Karmeli R (1998) Duplex scanning and CT angiography in the diagnosis of carotid artery occlusion: a prospective study. Eur J Vasc Endovasc Surg 16: 133–136

207. Lutsep H, ALbers G, de Crespigny A, Moseley M (1996) Diffusion Imaging of Human Stroke, Proceedings of the International Society for Magnetic Resonance in Medicine, 4th Scientific Meeting and Exhibition, New York, Vol 1

208. Lyden P, Brott T, Tilley B, Welch KM, Mascha EJ, Levine S, Haley EC, Grotta J, Marler J (1994) Improved reliability of the NIH Stroke Scale using video training. NINDS TPA Stroke Study Group. Stroke 25(11): 2220–2226

209. Lythgoe MF, Busza AL, Calamante F, Sotak CH, King MD, Bingham AC, Williams SR, Gadian DG (1997) Effects of diffusion anisotropy on lesion delineation in a rat model of cerebral ischemia. Magn Reson Med 38: 662–668

210. MacFall J, Prescott DM, Fullar E, Samulski TV (1995) Temperature dependence of canine

brain tissue diffusion coefficient measured in vivo with magnetic resonance echo-planar imaging. Int J Hyperthermia 11: 73–86

211. Mahoney FI, Barthel DW (1965) Functional Evaluation: The Barthel Index. Md Med J 21–23: 61–65

212. Manelfe C, Larrue V, von Kummer R, Bozzao L, Ringleb PA, Bastianello S, Iweins F, Lesaffre E (1999) Association of hyperdense middle cerebral artery sign with clinical outcome in patients treated with tissue plasminogen activator. Stroke 30(4): 769–772

213. Marks MP, Tong D, Beaulieu C, Albers G, de Crespigny A, Moseley ME (1999) Evaluation of early reperfusion and IV rt-PA therapy using diffusion- and perfusion-weighted MRI. Neurology 52: 1792–1798

214. Marler JR, Tilley BC, Lu M, Brott TG, Lyden PC, Grotta JC, Broderick JP, Levine SR, Frankel MP, Horowitz SH, Haley EC, Jr., Lewandowski CA, Kwiatkowski TP (2000) Early stroke treatment associated with better outcome: the NINDS rt-PA stroke study. Neurology 55(11): 1649–1655

215. Matsumoto K, Lo EH, Pierce AR, Wei H, Garrido L, Kowall NW (1995) Role of vasogenic edema and tissue cavitation in ischemic evolution on diffusion-weighted imaging: comparison with multiparameter MR and immunohistochemistry. AJNR Am J Neuroradiol 16: 1107–1115

216. Matsumura K, Matsuda M, Handa J, Todo G (1990) Magnetic resonance imaging with aneurysmal subarachnoid hemorrhage: comparison with computed tomography scan. Surg Neurol 34(2): 71–78

217. Mattle HP, Edelman RR, Schroth G, O'Reilly GV (1996) Spontaneous and Traumatic Hemorrhage in Clinical and Magnetic Resonance Imaging. Vol 1. Saunders, Philadelphia, pp 652–702

218. Melhem ER, Jara H, Eustace S (1997) Fluid-attenuated inversion recovery MR imaging: identification of protein concentration thresholds for CSF hyperintensity. AJR Am J Roentgenol 169(3): 859–862

219. Merboldt KD, Hänicke W, Bruhn H, Gyngell ML, Frahm J (1992) Diffusion imaging of the human brain in vivo using high-speed STEAM MRI. Magn Reson Med 23: 179–192

220. Merboldt KD, Hänicke W, Frahm J (1985) Self-diffusion NMR imaging using stimulated echoes. J Magn Reson 64: 479–486

221. Merboldt KD, Hänicke W, Gyngell ML, Frahm J, Bruhn H (1989) Rapid NMR imaging of molecular self diffusion using a modified CE FAST sequence. J Magn Reson 82: 115–121

222. Meyer JS, Gilroy J, Barnhart MI, Johnson JF (1963) Therapeutic thrombolysis in cerebral thromboembolism. Neurology 13: 927–937

223. Minematsu K, Hasegawa Y, Yamaguchi T (1995) Diffusion MRI for evaluating cerebrovascular disease. Rinsho Shinkeigaku 35(12): 1575–1577

224. Mintorovitch J, Moseley ME, Chileuitt L, Shimizu H, Cohen Y, Weinstein PR (1991) Comparison of diffusion- and T2-weighted MRI for the early detection of cerebral ischemia and reperfusion in rats. Magn Reson Med 18(1): 39–50

225. Mohr JP (2000) Thrombolytic therapy for ischemic stroke: from clinical trials to clinical practice. JAMA 283: 1189–1191

226. Mohr JP, Biller J, Hilal SK, Yuh WT, Tatemichi TK, Hedges S, Tali E, Nguyen H, Mun I, Adams HP, Jr., et al. (1995) Magnetic resonance versus computed tomographic imaging in acute stroke. Stroke 26(5): 807–812

227. Molina CA, Montaner J, Abilleira S, Arenillas JF, Ribo M, Huertas R, Romero F, Alvarez-Sabin J (2001) Time course of tissue plasminogen activator-induced recanalization in acute cardioembolic stroke: a case-control study. Stroke 32(12): 2821–2827

228. Molina CA, Montaner J, Abilleira S, Ibarra B, Romero F, Arenillas JF, Alvarez-Sabin J (2001) Timing of spontaneous recanalization and risk of hemorrhagic transformation in acute cardioembolic stroke. Stroke 32(5): 1079–1084

229. Moonis M, Fisher M (2001) Imaging of acute stroke. Cerebrovasc Dis 11: 143–150

230. Morgenstern LB, Frankowski RF, Shedden P, Pasteur W, Grotta JC (1998) Surgical Treatment for Intracerebral Hemorrhage (STICH). Stroke 51: 1359–1363

231. Mori E, Tabuchi M, Yoshida T, Yamadori A (1988) Intracarotid urokinase with thromboembolic occlusion of the middle cerebral artery. Stroke 19(7): 802–812

232. Mori E, Yoneda Y, Tabuchi M, Yoshida T, Ohkawa S, Ohsumi Y, Kitano K, Tsutsumi A, Yamadori A (1992) Intravenous recombinant tissue plasminogen activator in acute carotid artery territory stroke. Neurology 42(5): 976–982

233. Mori S, van Zijl PC (1995) Diffusion weighting by the trace of the diffusion tensor within a single scan. Magn Reson Med 33: 41–52

234. Morris AD, Ritchie C, Grosset DG, Adams FG, Lees KR (1995) A pilot study of streptokinase for acute cerebral infarction. QJM 88(10): 727–731

235. Moseley M (2000) Pathophysiologic Basis of Diffusion and Perfusion-Weighted Imaging, 25th International Stroke Conference, February 10th–12th, New Orleans, USA

236. Moseley ME, Kucharczyk J, Asgari HS, Norman D (1991) Anisotropy in diffusion-weighted MRI. Magn Reson Med 19(2): 321–326

237. Moseley ME, Kucharczyk J, Mintorovitch J, Cohen Y, Kurhanewicz J, Derugin N, Asgari H, Norman D (1990) Diffusion-weighted MR imaging of acute stroke: correlation with T2-weighted and magnetic susceptibility-enhanced MR imaging in cats. AJNR Am J Neuroradiol 11(3): 423–429

238. Moseley ME, Wendland MF, Kucharczyk J (1991) Magnetic resonance imaging of diffusion and perfusion. Top Magn Reson Imaging 3(3): 50–67

239. Mueller DP, Yuh WTC, Fisher DJ, Chandran KB, Crain MR, Kim YH (1993) Arterial enhancement in acute cerebral ischemia: clinical and angiographic correlation. AJNR Am J Neuroradiol 14: 661–668

240. Mun Bryce S, Kroh FO, White J, Rosenberg GA (1993) Brain lactate and pH dissociation in edema: 1H- and 31P-NMR in collagenase-induced hemorrhage in rats. Am J Physiol 265(3 Pt 2): R697–702

241. Neeman M, Freyer JP, Sillerud LO (1990) Pulsed-gradient spin-echo studies in NMR imaging. Effects of the imaging gradients on the determination of diffusion coefficients. J Magn Reson 90: 303–312

242. Neil JJ, Shiran SI, McKinstry RC, Schefft GL, Snyder AZ, Almli CR, Akbudak E, Aronovitz JA, Miller JP, Lee BC, Conturo TE (1998) Normal brain in human newborns: apparent diffusion coefficient and diffusion anisotropy measured by using diffusion tensor MR imaging. Radiology 209: 57–66

243. Neumann-Haefelin T, Kastrup A, de Crespigny A, Yenari MA, Ringer T, Sun GH, Moseley ME (2000) Serial MRI after transient focal cerebral ischemia in rats: dynamics of tissue injury, blood-brain barrier damage, and edema formation. Stroke 31(8): 1965–1972

244. Neumann-Haefelin T, Wittsack HJ, Wenserski F, Siebler M, Seitz RJ, Moedder U, Freund HJ (1999) Diffusion- and perfusion weighted MRI. The DWI/PWI mismatch region in acute stroke. Stroke 30: 1591–1597

245. Nighoghossian N, Berthezene Y, Meyer R, Cinotti L, Adeleine P, Philippon B, Froment JC, Trouillas P (1997) Assessment of cerebrovascular reactivity by dynamic susceptibility contrast-enhanced MR imaging. J Neurol Sci 149: 171–176

246. Nighoghossian N, Hermier M, Adeleine P, Blanc-Lasserre K, Derex L, Honnorat J, Philippeau F, Dugor JF, Froment JC, Trouillas P (2002) Old microbleeds are a potential risk factor for cerebral bleeding after ischemic stroke: a gradient-echo t2*-weighted brain MRI study. Stroke 33(3): 735–742

247. Noguchi K, Ogawa T, Inugami A, Toyoshima H, Okudera T, Uemura K (1994) MR of acute subarachnoid hemorrhage: a preliminary report of fluid-attenuated inversion-recovery pulse sequences. AJNR Am J Neuroradiol 15(10): 1940–1943

248. Noguchi K, Ogawa T, Inugami A, Toyoshima H, Sugawara S, Hatazawa J, Fujita H, Shimosegawa E, Kanno I, Okudera T, et al. (1995) Acute subarachnoid hemorrhage: MR imaging with fluid-attenuated inversion recovery pulse sequences. Radiology 196(3): 773–777

249. Noguchi K, Ogawa T, Seto H, Inugami A, Hadeishi H, Fujita H, Hatazawa J, Shimosegawa E, Okudera T, Uemura K (1997) Subacute and chronic subarachnoid hemorrhage: diagnosis with fluid-attenuated inversion-recovery MR imaging. Radiology 203(1): 257–262

250. Noguchi K, Seto H, Kamisaki Y, Tomizawa G, Toyoshima S, Watanabe N (2000) Comparison of fluid-attenuated inversion-recovery MR imaging with CT in a simulated model of acute subarachnoid hemorrhage. AJNR Am J Neuroradiol 21(5): 923–927

251. O'Connor RE, McGraw P, Edelsohn L (1999) Thrombolytic therapy for acute ischemic stroke: why the majority of patients remain ineligible for treatment. Ann Emerg Med 33: 9–14

252. Ogawa T, Inugami A, Shimosegawa E, Fujita H, Ito H, Toyoshima H, Sugawara S, Kanno I, Okudera T, Uemura K, et al. (1993) Subarachnoid hemorrhage: evaluation with MR imaging. Radiology 186(2): 345–351

253. Ohtomo E, Araki G, Itoh E, Toghi H, Matsuda T, Atarashi J (1985) Clinical efficacy of urokinase in the treatment of cerebral thrombosis. Multi-center double blind study in comparison with placebo (Translated from Japanese). Clin Eval 15(3): 711–731

254. Ono J, Harada K, Takahashi M, Maeda M, Ikenaka K, Sakurai K, Sakai N, Kagawa T, Fritz-Zieroth B, T TN (1995) Differentiation between dysmyelination and demyelination using magnetic resonance diffusional anisotropy. Brain Res 671: 141–148

255. Oppenheim C, Samson Y, Manai R, Lalam T, Vandamme X, Crozier S, Srour A, Cornu P, Dormont D, Rancurel G, Marsault C (2000) Prediction of malignant middle cerebral artery infarction by diffusion-weighted imaging. Stroke 31(9): 2175–2181

256. Osborn AG (1994) Intracranial hemorrhage. In: Osborn AG (ed) Diagnostic Neuroradiology, Mosby, Year Book Inc, pp 154–198

257. Ostergaard L, Weisskoff RM, Chesler DA, Gyldensted C, Rosen BR (1996) High resolution

measurement of cerebral blood flow using intravascular tracer bolus passages, part I: mathematical approach and statistical analysis. Magn Reson Med 36: 715–725

258. Parsons MW, Barber PA, Chalk J, Darby DG, Rose S, Desmond PM, Gerraty RP, Tress BM, Wright PM, Donnan GA, Davis SM (2002) Diffusion- and perfusion-weighted MRI response to thrombolysis in stroke. Ann Neurol 51(1): 28–37

259. Parsons MW, Barber PA, Davis SM (2002) Relationship between severity of MR perfusion deficit and DWI lesion evolution. Neurology 58(11): 1707; discussion 1707

260. Parsons MW, Yang Q, Barber PA, Darby DG, Desmond PM, Gerraty RP, Tress BM, Davis SM (2001) Perfusion magnetic resonance imaging maps in hyperacute stroke: relative cerebral blood flow most accurately identifies tissue destined to infarct. Stroke 32(7): 1581–1587

261. Patel MR, Edelman RR, Warach S (1996) Detection of hyperacute primary intraparenchymal hemorrhage by magnetic resonance imaging. Stroke 27(12): 2321–2324

262. Patel SC, Levine SR, Tilley BC, Grotta JC, Lu M, Frankel M, Haley EC, Jr., Brott TG, Broderick JP, Horowitz S, Lyden PD, Lewandowski CA, Marler JR, Welch KM (2001) Lack of clinical significance of early ischemic changes on computed tomography in acute stroke. JAMA 286(22): 2830–2838

263. Perthen JE, Calamante F, Gadian DG, Connelly A (2002) Is quantification of bolus tracking MRI reliable without deconvolution? Magn Res Med 47: 61–67

264. Pexman JH, Barber PA, Hill MD, Sevick RJ, Demchuk AM, Hudon ME, Hu WY, Buchan AM (2001) Use of the Alberta Stroke Program Early CT Score (ASPECTS) for assessing CT scans in patients with acute stroke. AJNR Am J Neuroradiol 22(8): 1534–1542

265. Pierce AR, Lo EH, Mandeville JB, Gonzalez RG, Rosen BR, Wolf GL (1997) MRI measurements of water diffusion and cerebral perfusion: their relationship in a rat model of focal cerebral ischemia. J Cereb Blood Flow Metab 17(2): 183–190

266. Pierpaoli C, Jezzard P, Basser PJ, Barnett A, Di Chiro G (1996) Diffusion tensor MR imaging of the human brain. Radiology 201: 637–648

267. Powers WJ (2000) Testing a test: a report card for DWI in acute stroke. Neurology 54(8): 1549–1551

268. Powers WJ, Zivin J (1998) Magnetic resonance imaging in acute stroke: not ready for prime time. Neurology 50(4): 842–843

269. Prasad PV, Nalcioglu O (1991) A modified pulse sequence for in vivo diffusion imaging with reduced motion artifacts. Magn Reson Med 18: 116–131

270. Provenzale JM, Engelter ST, Petrella JR, Smith JS, MacFall JR (1999) Use of MR exponential diffusion-weighted images to eradicate T2 "shine-through" effect. AJR Am J Roentgenol 172(2): 537–539

271. Quast MJ, Huang NC, Hillman GR, Kent TA (1993) The evolution of acute stroke recorded by multimodal magnetic resonance imaging. Magn Reson Imaging 11(4): 465–471

272. Rankin J (1957) Cerebral vascular accidents in people over the age of 60: prognosis. Scott Med J 2: 200–215

273. Reith W, Hasegawa Y, Latour LL, Dardzinski BJ, Sotak CH, Fisher M (1995) Multislice diffusion mapping for 3-D evolution of cerebral ischemia in a rat stroke model. Neurology 45: 172–177

274. Reith W, Heiland S, Erb G, Benner T, Forsting M, Sartor K (1997) Dynamic contrast-enhanced T2*-weighted MR imaging in patients with cerebrovascular disease. Neuroradiology 39: 250–257

275. Rempp KA, Brix G, Wenz F, Becker CR, Gückel F, Lorenz WJ (1994) Quantification of regional cerebral blood flow and volume with dynamic susceptibility contrast-enhanced MR imaging. Radiology 193: 637–641

276. Rieke K, Schwab S, Krieger D, von Kummer R, Aschoff A, Schuchardt V, Hacke W (1995) Decompressive surgery in space-occupying hemispheric infarction: results of an open, prospective trial. Crit Care Med 23(9): 1576–1587

277. Ringelstein EB, Biniek R, Weiller C, Ammeling B, Nolte PN, Thron A (1992) Type and extent of hemispheric brain infarctions and clinical outcome in early and delayed middle cerebral artery recanalization. Neurology 42(2): 289–298

278. Ringelstein EB, Schneider R, Koschorke S (1989) Analysis of patterns of hemispheric brain infarctions on CT: embolic stroke mechanism, territorial infarctions and lacunae. Psychiatry Res 29(3): 273–276

279. Roberts TP, Vexler Z, Derugin N, Moseley ME, Kucharczyk J (1993) High-speed MR imaging of ischemic brain injury following stenosis of the middle cerebral artery. J Cereb Blood Flow Metab 13: 940–946

280. Roberts TP, Vexler ZS, Vexler V, Derugin N, Kucharczyk J (1996) Sensitivity of high-speed 'perfusion-sensitive' magnetic resonance imaging to mild cerebral ischemia. Eur Radiol 6: 645–649

281. Rordorf G, Koroshetz WJ, Copen WA, Cramer SC, Schaefer PW, R F Budzik Jr, Schwamm LH, Buonanno F, Sorensen AG, Gonzalez G (1998) Regional ischemia and ischemic injury in pa-

tients with acute middle cerebral artery stroke as defined by early diffusion-weighted and perfusion-weighted MRI. Stroke 29: 939–943

282. Rordorf G, Koroshetz WJ, Copen WA, Gonzalez G, Yamada K, Schaefer PW, Schwamm LH, Ogilvy CS, Sorensen AG (1999) Diffusion- and perfusion-weighted imaging in vasospasm after subarachnoid hemorrhage. Stroke 30(3): 599–605

283. Rosen BR, Belliveau JW, Chien D (1989) Perfusion imaging by nuclear magnetic resonance. Magn Reson Q 5(4): 263–281

284. Rosen BR, Belliveau JW, Vevea JM, Brady TJ (1990) Perfusion imaging with NMR contrast agents. Magn Reson Med 14: 249–265

285. Rosenow F, Hojer C, Meyer-Lohmann C, Hilgers RD, Muhlhofer H, Kleindienst A, Owega A, Koning W, Heiss WD (1997) Spontaneous intracerebral hemorrhage. Prognostic factors in 896 cases. Acta Neurol Scand 96(3): 174–182

286. Röther J, de Crespigny AJ, Arceuil HD, Iwai K, Moseley ME (1996) Recovery of apparent diffusion coefficient after ischemia-induced spreading depression relates to cerebral perfusion gradient. Stroke 27(5): 980–986

287. Röther J, Gass A, Busch E (1999) Diffusion- and perfusion-weighted MRI in cerebral ischaemia – Part 1: results of animal experiments. Akt Neurol 26(7): 300–308

288. Röther J, Schellinger PD, Gass A, Siebler M, Villringer A, Fiebach JB, Fiehler J, Jansen O, Kucinski T, Schoder V, Szabo K, Junge-Hülsing GJ, Hennerici M, Zeumer H, Sartor K, Weiller C, Hacke W (2002) Effect of intravenous thrombolysis on MRI parameters and functional outcome in acute stroke <6 h. Stroke 33(10): 2438–2445

289. Ruiz-Sandoval JL, Cantu C, Barinagarrementeria F (1999) Intracerebral hemorrhage in young people: analysis of risk factors, location, causes, and prognosis. Stroke 30(3): 537–541

290. Runge VM, Kirsch JE, Lee C (1993) Contrast-enhanced MR angiography. J Magn Reson Imaging 3: 233–239

291. Runge VM, Kirsch JE, Wells JW, Woolfolk CE (1993) Assessment of cerebral perfusion by first-pass, dynamic, contrast-enhanced, steady-state free-precession MR imaging: an animal study. AJR Am J Roentgenol 160: 593–600

292. Sacco RL, DeRosa JT, Haley EC, Jr., Levin B, Ordronneau P, Phillips SJ, Rundek T, Snipes RG, Thompson JL (2001) Glycine antagonist in neuroprotection for patients with acute stroke: GAIN Americas: a randomized controlled trial. JAMA 285(13): 1719–1728

293. Sacco RL, Shi T, Zamanillo MC, Kargman DE (1994) Predictors of mortality and recurrence after hospitalized cerebral infarction in an urban community: The Northern Manhattan Stroke Study. Neurology 44: 626–634

294. Sager TN, Laursen H, Fink-Jensen A, Topp S, Stensgaard A, Hedehus M, Rosenbaum S, Valsborg JS, Hansen AJ (1999) N-Acetylaspartate distribution in rat brain striatum during acute brain ischemia. J Cereb Blood Flow Met 19(2): 164–172

295. Sartor K (2002) Diagnostic and Interventional Neuroradiology – A Multimodality Approach. Thieme, Stuttgart New York, pp 76, 141, 160–169

296. Sasaki O, Takeuchi S, Koike T, Koizumi T, Tanaka R (1995) Fibrinolytic therapy for acute embolic stroke: intravenous, intracarotid, and intra-arterial local approaches. Neurosurgery 36(2): 246–252

297. Satoh S, Kadoya S (1988) Magnetic resonance imaging of subarachnoid hemorrhage. Neuroradiology 30(5): 361–366

298. Saver JL, Johnston KC, Homer D, Wityk R, Koroshetz W, Truskowski LL, Haley EC (1999) Infarct Volume as a Surrogate or Auxiliary Outcome Measure in Ischemic Stroke Clinical Trials. Stroke 30: 293–298

299. Scandinavian Stroke Study Group (1985) Multicenter trial of hemodilution in ischemic stroke. Stroke 16: 885–890

300. Schaefer PW, Hassankhani A, Christopher R, Koroshetz WJ, Rordorf G, Schwamm LH, Buonanno F, Gonzalez RG (2002) Partial reversal of DWI abnormalities in stroke patients undergoing thrombolysis: evidence of DWI and ADC thresholds. Stroke 33(1): 357

301. Schellinger P, Steiner T (1998) Emergency and intensive-care treatment after a stroke. Recommendations of the European Consensus Group. Nervenarzt 69: 530–539

302. Schellinger PD, Fiebach JB, Jansen O, Ringleb PA, Mohr A, Steiner T, Heiland S, Schwab S, Pohlers O, Ryssel H, Orakcioglu B, Sartor K, Hacke W (2001) Stroke magnetic resonance imaging within 6 hours after onset of hyperacute cerebral ischemia. Ann Neurol 49(4): 460–469

303. Schellinger PD, Fiebach JB, Mohr A, Kollmar R, Schwarz S, Schäbitz WR, Sartor K, Hacke W (2001) The role of stroke MRI in intracranial and subarachnoid hemorrhage. Nervenarzt 72(12): 907–917

304. Schellinger PD, Fiebach JB, Mohr A, Ringleb PA, Jansen O, Hacke W (2001) Thrombolytic therapy for ischemic stroke – A review. Part II – Intra-arterial thrombolysis, vertebrobasilar stroke, phase IV trials, and stroke imaging. Crit Care Med 29(9): 1819–1825

305. Schellinger PD, Fiebach JB, Mohr A, Ringleb PA, Jansen O, Hacke W (2001) Thrombolytic therapy for ischemic stroke – A review. Part I

– Intravenous thrombolysis. Crit Care Med 29(9): 1812–1818

306. Schellinger PD, Jansen O, Fiebach JB, Hacke W, Sartor K (1999) A standardized MRI stroke protocol: comparison with CT in hyperacute intracerebral hemorrhage. Stroke 30: 765–768

307. Schellinger PD, Jansen O, Fiebach JB, Heiland S, Steiner T, Schwab S, Pohlers O, Ryssel H, Sartor K, Hacke W (2000) Monitoring intravenous recombinant tissue plasminogen activator thrombolysis for acute ischemic Stroke with diffusion and perfusion MRI. Stroke 31(6): 1318–1328

308. Schellinger PD, Jansen O, Fiebach JB, Pohlers O, Ryssel H, Heiland S, Steiner T, Hacke W, Sartor K (2000) Feasibility and practicality of MR imaging of stroke in the management of hyperacute cerebral ischemia. AJNR Am J Neuroradiol 21(7): 1184–1189

309. Schlaug G, Benfield A, Baird AE, Siewert B, Lovblad KO, Parker RA, Edelman RR, Warach S (1999) The ischemic penumbra: operationally defined by diffusion and perfusion MRI. Neurology 53(7): 1528–1537

310. Schmulling S, Grond M, Rudolf J, Heiss WD (2000) One-year follow-up in acute stroke patients treated with rtPA in clinical routine. Stroke 31(7): 1552–1554

311. Schramm P, Schellinger PD, Fiebach JB, Heiland S, Jansen O, Knauth M, Hacke W, Sartor K (2002) Comparison of CT and CT angiography source images with diffusion-weighted imaging in patients with acute stroke within 6 hours after onset. Stroke 33(10): 2426–2432

312. Schriger DL, Kalafut M, Starkman S, Krueger M, Saver JL (1998) Cranial computed tomography interpretation in acute stroke: physician accuracy in determining eligibility for thrombolytic therapy. JAMA 279(16): 1293–1297

313. Schwab S, Georgiadis D, Berrouschot J, Schellinger PD, Graffagnino C, Mayer SA (2001) Feasibility and safety of moderate hypothermia after massive hemispheric infarction. Stroke 32(9): 2033–2035

314. Schwab S, Schwarz S, Spranger M, Keller E, Bertram M, Hacke W (1998) Moderate hypothermia in the treatment of patients with severe middle cerebral artery infarction. Stroke 29: 2461–2466

315. Schwab S, Steiner T, Aschoff A, Schwarz S, Steiner HH, Jansen O, Hacke W (1998) Early hemicraniectomy in patients with complete middle cerebral artery infarction. Stroke 29: 1888–1893

316. Scotti G, Ethier R, Melancon D, Terbrugge K, Tchang S (1977) Computed tomography in the evaluation of intracranial aneurysms and subarachnoid hemorrhage. Radiology 123(1): 85–90

317. Shimosegawa E, Inugami A, Okudera T, Hatazawa J, Ogawa T, Fujita H, Toyoshima H, Uemura K (1993) Embolic cerebral infarction: MR findings in the first 3 hours after onset. Am J Roentgenol 160: 1077–1082

318. Shinar D, Gross CR, Hier DB, Caplan LR, Mohr JP, Price TR, Wolf PA, Kase CS, Fishman IG, Barwick JA, et al. (1987) Interobserver reliability in the interpretation of computed tomographic scans of stroke patients. Arch Neurol 44(2): 149–155

319. Shrier DA, Tanaka H, Numaguchi Y, Konno S, Patel U, Shibata D (1997) CT angiography in the evaluation of acute stroke. AJNR Am J Neuroradiol 18(6): 1011–1020

320. Slevin ML, Plant H, Lynch D, Drinkwater J, Gregory WM (1988) Who should measure quality of life, the doctor or the patient? Br J Cancer 57(1): 109–112

321. Sorensen AG (2001) What is the meaning of quantitative CBF? AJNR Am J Neuroradiol 22: 235–236

322. Sorensen AG, Buonanno FS, Gonzalez RG, Schwamm LH, Lev MH, Huang Hellinger FR, Reese TG, Weisskoff RM, Davis TL, Suwanwela N, Can U, Moreira JA, Copen WA, Look RB, Finklestein SP, Rosen BR, Koroshetz WJ (1996) Hyperacute stroke: evaluation with combined multisection diffusion-weighted and hemodynamically weighted echo-planar MR imaging. Radiology 199(2): 391–401

323. Stehling MK, Turner R, Mansfield P (1991) Echo-planar imaging: magnetic resonance imaging in a fraction of a second. Science 254: 43–50

324. Steinbrich W, Gross-Fengels W, Krestin GP, Heindel W, Schreier G (1990) Intracranial hemorrhages in the magnetic resonance tomogram. Studies on sensitivity, on the development of hematomas and on the determination of the cause of the hemorrhage. Rofo Fortschr Geb Rontgenstr Neuen Bildgeb Verfahr 152(5): 534–543

325. Steiner T, Bluhmki E, Kaste M, Toni D, Trouillas P, vonKummer R, Hacke W (1998) The ECASS 3-hour cohort. Secondary analysis of ECASS data by time stratification. Cerebrovasc Dis 8: 198–203

326. Steiner T, Hennes HJ, Ringleb P, Bertram M, Hacke W (1999) Zeitbasiertes Management des akuten Schlaganfalls. Notfall & Rettungsmedizin 2: 400–407

327. Stejskal EO, Tanner JE (1965) Spin diffusion measurements: spin echoes in the presence of a time-dependent field gradient. J Chem Phys 42: 288–292

328. Sunshine JL, Tarr RW, Lanzieri CF, Landis DMD, Selman WR, Lewin JS (1999) Hyperacute stroke: ultrafast MR imaging to triage

patients prior to therapy. Radiology 212: 325–332

329. Tanner JE, Stejskal EO (1968) Restricted self-diffusion of protons in colloidal systems by the pulsed-gradient, spin-echo method. Journal of Chemical Physics 49: 1768–1777

330. Teasdale G, Jannett B (1975) Assessment of outcome after severe brain damage. Lancet 1: 480–484

331. Teasdale G, Jennett B (1974) Assessment of coma and impaired consciousness. A practical scale. Lancet 2(7872): 81–84

332. The European Ad Hoc Consensus Group (1996) European strategies for early intervention in stroke. A report of an ad hoc consensus group meeting. Cerebrovasc Dis 6: 315–324

333. The European Ad Hoc Consensus Group (1997) Optimizing intensive care in stroke: a European perspective – a report of an Ad Hoc consensus group meeting. Cerebrovasc Dis 7: 113–128

334. The European Stroke Initiative (2000) Recommendations for stroke management. Cerebrovasc Dis 10(Suppl 3): 1–34

335. The GUSTO Angiographic Investigators (1993) The effects of tissue plasminogen activator, streptokinase or both on coronary artery patency, ventricular function, and survival after acute myocardial infarction. N Engl J Med 329: 1615–1622

336. The Multicenter Acute Stroke Trial–Europe Study Group (1996) Thrombolytic therapy with streptokinase in acute ischemic stroke. N Engl J Med 335(3): 145–150

337. The Multicentre Acute Stroke Trial–Italy (MAST-I) Group (1995) Randomised controlled trial of streptokinase, aspirin, and combination of both in treatment of acute ischaemic stroke. Lancet 346(8989): 1509–1514

338. The National Institute of Neurological Disorders and Stroke rt-PA Stroke Study Group (1995) Tissue plasminogen activator for acute ischemic stroke. N Engl J Med 333(24): 1581–1587

339. The TIMI Study Group (1985) The Thrombolysis in Myocardial Infarction (TIMI) trial. Phase I findings. N Engl J Med 312(14): 932–936

340. Theron J, Courtheoux P, Casasco A, Alachkar F, Notari F, Ganem F, Maiza D (1989) Local intraarterial fibrinolysis in the carotid territory. AJNR Am J Neuroradiol 10(4): 753–765

341. Tomsick T, Brott T, Barsan W, Broderick J, Haley EC, et al (1996) Prognostic value of the hyperdense middle cerebral artery sign and stroke scale score before ultraearly thrombolytic therapy. AJNR Am J Neuroradiol 17: 1–7

342. Tomsick TA, Brott TG, Chambers AA, Fox AJ, Caskill MF, Lukin RR, Pleatman CW, Wiot JG, Bourekas E (1990) Hyperdense middle cerebral artery sign on CT: efficacy in detecting middle cerebral artery thrombosis. AJNR Am J Neuroradiol 11(3): 473–477

343. Tomura N, Uemura K, Inugami A, Fujita H, Higano S, Shishido F (1988) Early CT finding in cerebral infarction: obscuration of the lentiform nucleus. Radiology 168(2): 463–467

344. Tong DC, Yenari MA, Albers GW, M OB, Marks MP, Moseley ME (1998) Correlation of perfusion- and diffusion-weighted MRI with NIHSS score in acute (<6.5 hour) ischemic stroke. Neurology 50(4): 864–870

345. Truwit CL, Barkovich AJ, Gean-Marton A, Hibri N, Norman D (1990) Loss of the insular ribbon: another early CT sign of acute middle cerebral artery infarction. Radiology 176(3): 801–806

346. Tsuchida C, Yamada H, Maeda M, Sadato N, Matsuda T, Kawamura Y, Hayashi N, Yamamoto K, Yonekura Y, Ishii Y (1997) Evaluation of peri-infarcted hypoperfusion with T2*-weighted dynamic MRI. J Magn Reson Imaging 7: 518–522

347. Turner R, Le Bihan D, Maier J, Vavrek R, Hedges LK, Pekar J (1990) Echo-planar imaging of intravoxel incoherent motion. Radiology 177: 407–414

348. Turner R, von Kienlin M, Moonen CT, van Zijl PC (1990) Single-shot localized echo-planar imaging (STEAM-EPI) at 4.7 tesla. Magn Reson Med 14: 401–408

349. Ueda T, Hatakeyama T, Kumon Y, Sakaki S, Uraoka T (1994) Evaluation of risk of hemorrhagic transformation in local intra-arterial thrombolysis in acute ischemic stroke by initial SPECT. Stroke 25(2): 298–303

350. Ueda T, Sakaki S, Kumon Y, Ohta S (1999) Multivariable analysis of predictive factors related to outcome at 6 months after intra-arterial thrombolysis for acute ischemic stroke. Stroke 30(11): 2360–2365

351. Ueda T, Sakaki S, Yuh WT, Nochide I, Ohta S (1999) Outcome in acute stroke with successful intra-arterial thrombolysis and predictive value of initial single-photon emission-computed tomography. J Cereb Blood Flow Metab 19(1): 99–108

352. van Everdingen KJ, van der Grond J, Kappelle LJ, Ramos LMP, Mali WPTM (1998) Diffusion-weighted magnetic resonance imaging in acute stroke. Stroke 29: 1783–1790

353. van Gelderen P, de Vleeschouwer MH, DesPres D, Pekar J, van Zijl PC, Moonen CT (1994) Water diffusion and acute stroke. Magn Reson Med 31(2): 154–163

354. van Gijn J (1992) Measurement of outcome in stroke prevention trials. Cerebrovasc Dis 2(Suppl 1): 23–24

355. van Gijn J, van Dongen KJ (1982) The time course of aneurysmal haemorrhage on computed tomograms. Neuroradiology 23(3): 153–156

356. Vexler ZS, Roberts TP, Bollen AW, Derugin N, Arieff AJ (1997) Transient cerebral ischemia. Association of apoptosis induction with hypoperfusion. J Clin Invest 99: 1453–1459

357. Videen TO, Dunford-Shore JE, Diringer MN, Powers WJ (1999) Correction for partial volume effects in regional blood flow measurements adjacent to hematomas in humans with intracerebral hemorrhage: implementation and validation. J Comput Assist Tomogr 23(2): 248–256

358. Villringer A, Rosen BR, Belliveau JW, Ackerman JL, Lauffer RB, Buxton RB, Chao YS, Wedeen VJ, Brady TJ (1988) Dynamic imaging with lanthanide chelates in normal rat brain: contrast due to magnetic susceptibility effects. Magn Reson Med 6: 164 –174

359. Vogl TJ, Heinzinger K, Juergens M, Kutter R, Hepp W, Balzer JO, Haupt G, Banzer D, Felix R (1995) Multiple slab MR angiography of the A. carotis interna: a preoperative comparative study. Rofo Fortschr Geb Rontgenstr Neuen Bildgeb Verfahr 162: 404–411

360. von Kummer R (1998) Effect of training in reading CT scans on patient selection for ECASS II. Neurology 51(3 Suppl 3): S50–S52

361. von Kummer R, Allen KL, Holle R, Bozzao L, Manelfe SB, Bluhmki E, Ringleb PA, Meier DH, Hacke W (1997) Acute stroke: usefulness of early CT findings before thrombolytic therapy. Radiology 205(2): 327–333

362. von Kummer R, Berrouschot J, Barthel H, Hesse S, Dieler C, Schneider D (2000) The effect of early and late brain tissue reperfusion on infarct volume (Abstract). Stroke 31: 275

363. von Kummer R, Bourquain H, Bastianello S, Bozzao L, Manelfe C, Meier D, Hacke W (2001) Early prediction of irreversible brain damage after ischemic stroke at CT. Radiology 219(1): 95–100

364. von Kummer R, Bozzao L, Manelfe C (1995) Early CT Diagnosis of Hemispheric Brain Infarction. Springer, Berlin, pp :1–95

365. von Kummer R, Gahn G (2000) Comparison of diffusion-weighted MRI and CT in acute stroke. Neurology 55(11): 1760

366. von Kummer R, Holle R, Gizyska U, Hofmann E, Jansen O, Petersen D, Schumacher M, Sartor K (1996) Interobserver agreement in assessing early CT signs of middle cerebral artery infarction. Am J Neuroradiol 17(9): 1743–1748

367. von Kummer R, Holle R, Rosin L, Forsting M, Hacke W (1995) Does arterial recanalization improve outcome in carotid territory stroke? Stroke 26(4): 581–587

368. von Kummer R, Meyding-Lamade U, Forsting M, Rosin L, Rieke K, Hacke W, Sartor K (1994) Sensitivity and prognostic value of early CT in occlusion of the middle cerebral artery trunk. Am J Neuroradiol 15(1): 9–15

369. von Kummer R, Nolte PN, Schnittger H, Thron A, Ringelstein EB (1996) Detectability of cerebral hemisphere ischaemic infarcts by CT within 6 h of stroke. Neuroradiology 38(1): 31–33

370. Warach S (2001) Tissue viability thresholds in acute stroke: the 4-factor model. Stroke 32(11): 2460–2461

371. Warach S, Boska M, Welch KM (1997) Pitfalls and potential of clinical diffusion-weighted MR imaging in acute stroke. Stroke 28(3): 481–482

372. Warach S, Chien D, Li W, Ronthal M, Edelman RR (1992) Fast magnetic resonance diffusion-weighted imaging of acute human stroke. Neurology 42(9): 1717–1723

373. Warach S, Dashe JF, Edelman RR (1996) Clinical outcome in ischemic stroke predicted by early diffusion-weighted and perfusion magnetic resonance imaging: a preliminary analysis. J Cereb Blood Flow Metab 16(1): 53–59

374. Warach S, Hacke W, Hsu C, Luby M, Sullivan M, Noonan T (2002) Effect of maxipost on ischemic lesions in patients with acute stroke: the POST-010 MRI substudy. Stroke 33: 383

375. Warach S, Kaste M, Fisher M (2000) The effect of GV150526 on ischemic lesion volume: the GAIN Americas and GAIN International MRI Substudy. Neurology 54(suppl3): A87–A88

376. Warach S, Li W, Ronthal M, Edelman RR (1992) Acute cerebral ischemia: evaluation with dynamic contrast-enhanced MR imaging and MR angiography. Radiology 182: 41–47

377. Warach S, Pettigrew LC, Dashe JF, Pullicino P, Lefkowitz DM, Sabounjian L, Harnett K, Schwiderski U, Gammans R (2000) Effect of citicoline on ischemic lesions as measured by diffusion-weighted magnetic resonance imaging. Citicoline 010 Investigators. Ann Neurol 48(5): 713–722

378. Warach S, Sabounjian LA (2000) ECCO 2000 study of citicoline for treatment of acute ischemic stroke: effects on infarct volumes measured by MRI. Stroke 31(1): 42

379. Wardlaw JM, del Zoppo G, Yamaguchi T (2002) Thrombolysis for acute ischaemic stroke (Cochrane Review) The Cochrane Library. Vol. Issue 1

380. Wardlaw JM, Sandercock PA, Warlow CP, Lindley RI (2000) Trials of thrombolysis in acute

ischemic stroke: does the choice of primary outcome measure really matter? Stroke 31(5): 1133–1135

381. Weber J, Reith W, Heiland S, Benner T, Dörfler A, Forsting M, Sartor K (1997) Computed tomography, perfusion and diffusion-weighted magnetic resonance imaging: Which method detects cerebral ischemia first?, ISMRM, Fifth Scientific Meeting, Vol. Book of Abstracts

382. Weingarten K, Zimmerman RD, Cahill PT, Deck MD (1991) Detection of acute intracerebral hemorrhage on MR imaging: ineffectiveness of prolonged interecho interval pulse sequences. AJNR Am J Neuroradiol 12(3): 475–479

383. Weisskoff RM, Chesler D, Boxerman JL, Rosen BR (1993) Pitfalls in MR measurements of tissue blood flow with intravascular tracers: which mean transit time? Magn Reson Med 29: 553–559

384. Welch KMA, Windham J, Knight RA, Nagesh V, Hugg JW, Jacobs M, Peck D, Booker P, Dereski MO, Levine SR (1995) A Model to Predict the Histopathology of Human Stroke Using Diffusion and T2-Weighted Magnetic Resonance Imaging. Stroke 26(11): 1983–1989

385. Wenz F, Baudendistel K, Wildermuth S, Heß T, Egelhof T, Forsting M, Schad LR, Knopp MV (1995) Quantification of the hemispheric asymmetry during finger movement using functional magnetic resonance imaging. Klinische Neuroradiologie 5(2): 53–60

386. WHO Guidelines Subcommittee (1999) 1999 World Health Organization-International Society of Hypertension Guidelines for the Management of Hypertension. J Hypertens 17(2): 151–183

387. WHO Task Force (1989) Recommendations on stroke prevention, diagnosis, and therapy. Report of the WHO Task Force on Stroke and other Cerebrovascular Disorders. Stroke 20(10): 1407–1431

388. Wiesmann M, Mayer TE, Medele R, Bruckmann H (1999) Diagnosis of acute subarachnoid hemorrhage at 1.5 Tesla using proton-density weighted FSE and MRI sequences. Radiologe 39(10): 860–865

389. Wildermuth S, Knauth M, Brandt T, Winter R, Sartor K, Hacke W (1998) Role of CT angiography in patient selection for thrombolytic therapy in acute hemispheric stroke. Stroke 29(5): 935–938

390. Yamada K, Wu O, Gonzalez RG, Bakker D, Østergaard L, Copen WA, Weisskoff RM, Rosen BR, Yagi K, Nishimura T, Sorensen AG (2002) Magnetic resonance perfusion-weighted imaging of acute cerebral infarction: effect of the calculation methods and underlying vasculopathy. Stroke 33(1): 87–94

391. Yamaguchi T, Hayakawa T, Kiuchi H, Japanese Thrombolysis Study Group (1993) Intravenous tissue plasminogen activator ameliorates the outcome of hyperacute embolic stroke. Cerebrovasc Dis 3: 269–272

392. Yuh WTC, Crain MR, Loes DJ, Greene GM, Ryals TJ, Sato Y (1991) MR imaging of cerebral ischemia: findings in the first 24 hours. AJNR Am J Neuroradiol 12: 621–629

393. Zazulia AR, Diringer MN, Videen TO, Adams RE, Yundt K, Aiyagari V, Grubb RL, Jr., Powers WJ (2001) Hypoperfusion without ischemia surrounding acute intracerebral hemorrhage. J Cereb Blood Flow Metab 21(7): 804–810

394. Zeumer H (1985) Vascular recanalizing technique in interventional neuroradiology. J Neurol 231: 287–294

395. Zeumer H, Freitag HJ, Zanella F, Thie A, Arning C (1993) Local intra-arterial fibrinolytic therapy in patients with stroke: urokinase versus recombinant tissue plasminogen activator (r-TPA). Neuroradiology 35(2): 159–162

396. Zierler KL (1962) Theoretical basis of indicator-dilution methods for measuring flow and volume. Circ Res 10: 393–407

397. Zivin JA, Holloway RG (2000) Weighing the evidence on DWI: caveat emptor. Neurology 54(8): 1552

398. Zyed A, Hayman LA, Bryan RN (1991) MR imaging of intracerebral blood: diversity in the temporal pattern at 0.5 and 1.0 T. AJNR Am J Neuroradiol 12(3): 469–474

Subject Index